OUTPATIENT ANESTHESIA

OUTPATIENT ANESTHESIA

CONTEMPORARY ANESTHESIA PRACTICE

BURNELL R. BROWN, JR., EDITOR

F. A. DAVIS COMPANY / PHILADELPHIA

Second printing 1979

Printed in the United States of America.

Library of Congress Cataloging in Publication Data
Main entry under title:

Outpatient anesthesia.

(Contemporary anesthesia practice ; 1)
Includes bibliographical references and index.
1. Anesthesia. 2. Surgery, Outpatient. I. Brown, Burnell R. II. Series.
RD82.087 617'.96 78-14424
ISBN 0-8036-1256-7

PREFACE

The CONTEMPORARY ANESTHESIA PRACTICE series is designed to present to the practicing anesthesiologist recent developments in clinical anesthesia care in a practical and meaningful form. The approach will be one of "how to do it" and "what we observed" in specific areas of care.

Outpatient Anesthesia, first in the series, deals with surgery on one-day basis, that is, ambulatory surgery. The facilities and personnel, economics, patient selection and care, techniques, and drug selection are thoroughly discussed. Also, the treatment of acute and chronic pain on an outpatient basis is covered. Our experiences with ambulatory surgery are primarily the result of work at the Ambulatory Surgery Center at Tucson Medical Center.

I am grateful to the individual authors for their excellent contributions to this first volume.

Burnell R. Brown, Jr.

CONTRIBUTORS

Lawrence Adler, M.D.
Associate Professor of Anesthesiology
University of Arizona College of Medicine
Tucson, Arizona

Casey Blitt, M.D.
Associate Professor of Anesthesiology
University of Arizona College of Medicine,
Tucson, Arizona

Burnell R. Brown, Jr., M.D., Ph.D.
Professor and Chairman
Department of Anesthesiology
University of Arizona College of Medicine
Tucson, Arizona

M. Lawrence Cobb, M.D.
Associate Professor
Department of Anesthesia
Washington University School of Medicine
St. Louis, Missouri

James B. Duckett, M.D. *(Deceased)*
Assistant Professor
Department of Anesthesiology
University of Texas Southwestern Medical School
Director, Day Surgery Unit
Parkland Memorial Hospital
Dallas, Texas

Lloyd Epstein, M.D.
Department of Surgery
Tucson Medical Center
Tucson, Arizona

Lawrence Haas, M.D.
Associate in Surgery (Orthopedics)
University of Arizona College of Medicine
Tucson, Arizona

Donald E. Howland, M.D.
Associate in Anesthesiology
University of Arizona College of Medicine
Tucson, Arizona

Laurel Ann Howland, R.N.
Research Assistant to Donald E. Howland, M.D.
Surgicenter®
Phoenix, Arizona

Fred H. Landeen, M.D.
Associate in Anesthesiology
University of Arizona College of Medicine
Tucson, Arizona

Larry P. Putnam, M.D.
Associate in Anesthesiology
University of Arizona College of Medicine
Tucson, Arizona

Wallace A. Reed, M.D.
Co-Director, Surgicenter®
Phoenix, Arizona

C. Ronald Stephen, M.D.
Professor and Chairman
Department of Anesthesia
Washington University School of Medicine
St. Louis, Missouri

CONTENTS

III

OUTPATIENT ANESTHESIA AT THE AMBULATORY SURGERY CENTER, TUCSON MEDICAL CENTER

Larry P. Putnam, M.D., and
Fred H. Landeen, M.D.

Drs. Putnam and Landeen are private practitioners with an interest in outpatient anesthesia. The Ambulatory Surgery Center at Tucson Medical Center is a model of economy, patient convenience, and efficient use of time. As an observer in this facility, one is impressed by the safe and deft handling of cases; patient recovery time is greatly reduced. Surgeons and patients alike are well satisfied with this dynamic clinic. The first chapter describes, in contrast to the freestanding Surgicenter[R] concept, an outpatient surgical facility created by a community hospital.

Burnell R. Brown, Jr.

HISTORY

Ambulatory surgical care is by no means a new or modern-day discovery. It might be more appropriate to say that it has been rediscovered.

One of the earliest reports of outpatient surgical care was made in 1909 by Nicole of Glasgow, in the British Medical Journal. He reported 8,988 surgical procedures safely performed on children as outpatients that led him to comment that "experience of herniotomy, abdominal section and other operations in young children treated as outpatients is gradually reconciling me to the view that we keep similar cases in adults too long in bed."[1]

One of the first to champion the concept in the United States was a physician known for many other contributions to the field of anesthesiology, among them the introduction of cyclopropane into clinical practice in 1934. Dr. Ralph M. Waters described his activity in this field in 1919 in a paper entitled *The down-town anesthesia clinic,* which appeared in the anesthesia supplement of the American Journal of Surgery. He described his clinic: "In our operating room. . . . we have a modified French chair-table [which]. . . . we find very convenient for the dentists' use. . . . it also makes an excellent flat operating table. We also have a dental engine, a sink with foot pedals to turn on water and a sterilizer for instruments, gauze, towels, gowns, et cetera, and a sterile water tank. In short, the usual equipment for a minor surgery room."[2]

The AMA, approving Resolution 33 in 1971, officially endorsed the safety of outpatient surgery when patients are carefully screened. Resolution 33 recognized that outpatient surgery under selected circumstances is a part of good medical practice.

CONCEPT

Today, surgery without overnight hospital stay is performed with increasing frequency all over the country. It is variously termed ambulatory surgery, short stay surgery, in-and-out surgery, outpatient surgery, and day surgery. Whatever the nomenclature, this type can be characterized as uncomplicated surgery that has been done in hospital but can be done equally well outside.

It has been estimated that 20 percent of all surgical procedures performed in hospital would be performed as successfully on an outpatient basis.[3]

Ambulatory surgery is not to be categorized with minor surgical procedures performed in surgeons' offices, emergency rooms, or in operating rooms under local anesthesia. Ambulatory surgery denotes more significant procedures, usually requiring general anesthesia and/or a period of postoperative observation. It has been shown, however, that this group of patients do not require, nor do they derive benefit from, the customary inpatient stay.

BENEFITS

Numerous in-depth studies have documented the savings in terms of both hospital expenses and hospital beds afforded by this method of surgical care. The benefits are enjoyed by all parties: the patient, the surgeon, the third party insurance carriers, and the hospital.

The daily hospital service charge represents the largest single expense saved in outpatient day surgery. (There is no difference in operating and recovery room and anesthesia supply costs). Ambulatory surgery results in an average 25 percent reduction in hospital charges, and a bed utilization savings of about 2 bed-days per patient. The patient's daily routine and schedule, and that of his family, are less disrupted, and his medical expenses are lower. The surgeon's time is used more economically. Third party carriers benefit directly from the reduction in hospital expense, and also from the elimination of the "nonessential" tests and services that sometimes accrue to the inpatient. The hospital administration is able to serve a larger population and to utilize more efficiently its expensive investments in operating suites, recovery areas, and anesthesia services.[4]

TYPES OF FACILITIES

Ambulatory surgery is performed in various parts of the country in several different ways. The facilities are classified in either of two general categories: (a) hospital-associated, or (b) freestanding.

Of the hospital-associated units, several different physical arrangements are being utilized: a *special ward* for admission, preoperative evaluation, and postoperative observation, with use of the existing hospital operating suites and recovery areas; *utilization of the existing recovery area,* for admission, preoperative screening, and postoperative care, with operative procedures carried out in the existing operating rooms; and the *autonomous unit,* with its own operating suite and preoperative and postoperative care facilities.

The freestanding unit provides preoperative, intraoperative, and postoperative care and is neither contained within nor attached to another health care facility. The Surgicenter[R] in Phoenix is the prototype of this type of facility.

AMBULATORY SURGERY CENTER, TUCSON MEDICAL CENTER

The Ambulatory Surgery Center at Tucson Medical Center (TMC) opened its doors to patients in February of 1974. It was created for the purpose of providing the TMC medical staff and Tucson, and surrounding communities, with an adequately staffed and organized facility in which surgical procedures can be safely carried out on a one-day basis. The unit is operated in strict accordance with the standards of TMC, The Associated Hospital Service of Arizona, and the JCAH. The unit is a department of TMC and reports to the hospital administrator or his designee. Medical direction is given by an anesthesiologist (title, Medical Director) assigned full-time to the unit. The Ambulatory Surgery Center at TMC is a hospital-based unit of the autonomous type containing 4 operating rooms, a 12-bed adult and 2-bed pediatric recovery area, 4 preoperative preparation and examining rooms, a reception area, and a waiting room area with an attached open-air patio.

Surgical Privileges

Surgeons who wish to utilize the Center must be members of the TMC medical staff. Their privileges are delineated within their respective surgical specialties. Anesthesiologists administering anesthesia in the unit must be members of the medical staff, and have privileges as delineated within their specialty.

Patient Selection Criteria

Each surgeon who schedules cases in the unit is responsible for scheduling patients who meet the criteria established by the Ambulatory Surgical Care committee. Surgical procedures must be on the list of those approved by the committee as safe to perform on outpatients and requiring not more than 8 hours' recovery time. Only patients falling into the American Society of Anesthesiologists (ASA) physical status categories I and II are accepted. Preadmission laboratory work must fall within acceptable limits and be performed within 72 hours prior to the scheduled procedure by the hospital lab or an accredited outside lab. A history and physical examination must be performed on each patient by the surgeon or by a qualified physician chosen by the surgeon. The Medical Director or his designee has the final responsibility for screening each patient prior to the procedure to insure that lab work, history, and physical and general patient evaluation indicate acceptability. It is his responsibility to cancel an unacceptable case and notify the attending surgeon of his findings. Due to the nature of the unit, *no chances are taken.*

Operating Room Schedule

The Center operates on a 5-day week, Monday through Friday, from 7:30 AM to 5:00 PM. Cases begin at 7:30 and run on a "to-follow" basis thereafter. Cases are not generally begun after 1:30 PM. Emergency cases are accepted if time is available on the schedule and if the procedure is one permitted in the unit and all other criteria are met.

Scheduling Procedure

Cases are scheduled for surgeons by their secretarial staffs. A single telephone call arranges anesthesia coverage and operating time. If there is sufficient time, written instructions are mailed to the patient. Otherwise, instructions are given to the patient by the surgeon and again by telephone call from the Center secretaries before the scheduled procedure.

Upon patient arrival at the facility, a chart is begun by the receptionist. The patient is taken to an examining room to change into a disposable gown and paper foot covers. The nurse in charge of patient admissions then asks pertinent questions to elicit the patient's previous medical history and experience with anesthesia. Temperature and blood pressure are taken, a lab technician obtains blood for hemoglobin and hematocrit and occasionally for potassium, and urine specimen is collected for urinalysis. Oral antacid tablets are also given at this time to those patients about to undergo general anesthesia.

Next, the anesthesiologist reviews the medical history, interviews the patient, and performs a physical examination of the heart and lungs. If in the course of examination it is noted that the patient has not complied with all NPO restrictions, has fever or a recently acquired upper respiratory infection, or if there is any contraindication to the proposed procedure, the anesthesiologist notifies the surgeon of his findings and outlines corrective measures. The patient is informed that the procedure must be postponed.

Premedication is given routinely only to those patients undergoing procedures under local anesthesia. Other patients are given reading material and encouraged to relax and listen to music while waiting for their surgeon to arrive. When the surgeon arrives, the patient is again identified after exchange of amenities and transported to the operating suite. This arrangement allows for last-minute questions or instructions to the patient by the surgeon and allows the patient to wait in relaxed, quiet surroundings, rather than in the operating room.

A tape cassette attached to a clip board with the record accompanies the patient from the time of admission to the unit until he is discharged from the recovery area. A cassette recorder is available in each operating room, so that the surgeon can dictate the operative report at the end of the procedure while he is still in the operating room. After checking the tape playback the surgeon signs the record and, except for an occasional prescription or list of patient instructions, no other record-keeping is required of him. The anesthesiologist completes the anesthesia part of the record. If circumstances warrant additional information, he may also dictate on the cassette for transcription into the record. This simple method obviates reams of incomplete charts awaiting the surgeon or anesthesiologist in the records room.

After completion of the procedure, the patient is taken to the recovery area to be cared for by a staff of experienced recovery room nurses. As soon as the patient is able to tolerate fluids, coffee, tea, or soft drinks are encouraged.

When recovery is sufficient, patients are allowed to sit on the bedside and then to ambulate with assistance to the bathroom. They are transferred to a wheelchair and allowed to remain seated for transfer to their automobiles. An anesthesiologist remains in the area until the last patient of the day has been given a final check and released. Patients are transported by wheelchair a short distance to a drive-through covered area where they are discharged to the care of a responsible adult to be driven home.

At the time of discharge, the patient is reminded of the surgeon's postoperative orders and given any appropriate prescriptions. He is reminded not to drive, sign any important papers, or make any important decisions for the remainder of the 24-hour period. A Center nurse calls each patient for a follow-up check.

The Costs–Charge Formula

The normal charge for the ambulatory surgery procedure at TMC is based on the estimated time that a patient will be in the operating room suite:

30 minutes or less	95.00
31 minutes to 45 minutes	135.00
each additional 15 minutes	25.00

(Includes 2.50 for CS supplies, 6.00 for laboratory, 3.00 for disposables.)

Sample Procedure Fees:

Bartholin cystectomy	$ 95.00
Cervical conization	135.00
D and C	95.00
Abortion	95.00
Laparoscopy	160.00

Other Center Charges:

Recovery room only	$ 30.00
Operating room only	
30 minutes or less	60.00

Total Facility Charge for Procedure Includes:

1. Use of operating room and recovery area
2. Medications
3. Materials
4. Laboratory tests
5. Operating microscope
6. Electrosurgical unit
7. Sterile supplies
8. Intravenous fluids
9. Local or general anesthesia supplies

Additional Charges:

1. Surgeon's fee
2. Anesthesiologist's fee
3. Pathologist's fee for frozen sections, specimens

Results by Year

1974 (February through December)

Total Procedures	3,616
Types of Procedures	
Excisions	876
D and C	665
Laparoscopy	399
Myringotomy	108
Herniorrhaphy	148
Abortions	293
Myringotomy, adenoidectomy	106
Tooth extraction	50
Marsupialization	31
Carpal tunnel release	29
Cryohemorrhoidectomy	119
Sigmoidoscopy	22
Biopsy	125
Strabismus	14
Fissurectomy	20
Tonsillectomy, adenoidectomy	5
Cystoscopy	16
Laryngoscopy	7
Other (e.g., examinations under anesthesia, manipulations)	552

1975	
Total Procedures	4,055
Types of Procedures	
Excisions	985
D and C	756
Laparoscopy	444
Myringotomy	128
Herniorrhaphy	162
Abortions	317
Myringotomy, adenoidectomy	118
Tooth extraction	52
Marsupialization	31
Carpal tunnel release	29
Cryohemorrhoidectomy	134
Circumcision	37
Sigmoidoscopy	22
Biopsy	148
Strabismus	15
Fissurectomy	20
Tonsillectomy, adenoidectomy	5
Cystoscopy	20
Laryngoscopy	7
Other (e.g., examinations under anesthesia, manipulations)	624

1976	
Total Procedures	5,606
Types of Procedures	
Excisions	1,056
D and C	1,005
Laparoscopy	975
Myringotomy	208
Herniorrhaphy	118
Abortions	307
Myringotomy, adenoidectomy	119
Tooth extraction	63
Marsupialization	13
Carpal tunnel release	15
Cryohemorrhoidectomy	113
Circumcision	44

Sigmoidoscopy	1
Biopsy	242
Strabismus	21
Fissurectomy	9
Tonsillectomy, adenoidectomy	5
Cystoscopy	221
Laryngoscopy	34
Other (e.g., examinations under anesthesia, manipulations)	998

1977 (through June)	
Total Procedures	3,370
Types of Procedures	
Excisions	338
D and C	497
Laparoscopy	655
Myringotomy	138
Herniorrhaphy	87
Abortions	185
Myringotomy, adenoidectomy	93
Tooth extraction	50
Marsupialization	0
Carpal tunnel release	39
Cryohemorrhoidectomy	64
Circumcision	30
Sigmoidoscopy	28
Biopsy	168
Strabismus	21
Fissurectomy	2
Tonsillectomy, adenoidectomy	0
Cystoscopy	155
Laryngoscopy	19
Other (e.g., examinations under anesthesia, manipulations	761

Procedures by Specialty	*1974*	*1975*	*1976*	*1977* (through June)
Ob-Gyn	1,378	1,538	2,301	2,099
General surgery	1,349	1,507	1,726	1,264
ENT	232	265	347	360
Orthopedics	175	192	285	273

Pediatric surgery	150	162	121	163
Eye	77	100	167	141
Dental	47	49	62	68
Plastics	157	180	292	256
Urology	49	60	284	269
Neurosurgery	0	2	21	100
Vascular	0	0	0	1

ANESTHETIC TECHNIQUES FOR AMBULATORY SURGERY

Anesthesia for ambulatory surgical procedures falls into three categories: (1) local anesthesia administered by the operating surgeon; (2) general anesthesia; (3) regional anesthesia administered by an anesthesiologist.

Local Anesthesia

These patients are premedicated in the examination rooms by the surgeon with drugs of his choice. They are monitored by a nurse intraoperatively, the extent dependent upon the surgeon's wishes. They are kept in the recovery room long enough to recover from the effects of their premedication, then allowed to go home in a manner similar to that of patients receiving general anesthesia.

General Anesthesia

General anesthetic techniques for the ambulatory patient are, of course, tailored to provide the operative conditions and permit the patient to awaken quickly and to fully regain his mental and physical capabilities as rapidly as possible with minimum side effects. Reed, at the Surgicenter[R] in Phoenix, describes a term he coined, *paramalgesia,* which consists of *para*lysis from a muscle relaxant drug, *am*nesia from 150 to 250 mg of a barbiturate such as thiamylal sodium (Surital) and anal*gesia* from N_2O - O_2 (3:1). They supplement this paramalgesic base with Meperidine or Fentanyl or with small amounts of volatile agents such as halothane or enflurane.[5] The Center at TMC utilizes somewhat similar techniques. Methohexital is used as an induction agent in 80- to 100-mg doses of methohexital and 0.1 percent succinylcholine if needed.

Laparoscopy and tubal coagulation is one of the most frequently performed procedures at the Center. The anesthetic technique utilized is fairly typical of that used for most other operations. After placement on the patient of a blood pressure cuff and a Space Labs telemetry monitor, an intravenous route is established and approximately 100 mg of Brevital is administered for induction. Anesthesia is maintained with enflurane in oxygen plus succinylcholine 0.1 percent drip as needed for relaxation. No more than 3 liters of CO_2 is insufflated for production of pneumoperitoneum and only mild Trendelenburg position is used. In the absence of other indications, the trachea is not usually intubated. The average time from cannula insertion for CO_2 insufflation to skin closure is less than 20 minutes, with the average anesthesia time around 20 to 25 minutes. There is no hesitation to intubate the trachea of anyone with airway maintenance problems, obesity, or any other condition which makes any other management unsafe.

Most procedures in adults are done with methohexital, O_2-enflurane-N_2O, succinylcholine drip sequence, while halothane is occasionally used. Most children receive inhalation inductions with N_2O, O_2 and halothane and are maintained with O_2, N_2O, and halothane.

Regional Anesthesia

Regional anesthesia at the Center at TMC is mostly limited to intravenous regional blocks and to perirectal blocks for anorectal procedures. Intravenous regional anesthesia is utilized for its simplicity, predictability, and relative rapidity of establishment of effect. It is used for most hand procedures, ganglionectomy, and carpal tunnel release.

Anesthesia for anorectal procedures done on ambulatory patients brings a special set of considerations. We are faced with a need for dependable anesthesia, technically easy to administer and allowing rapid recovery with minimum side effects. Conventional regional anesthesia such as hypobaric or hyperbaric subarachnoid block, epidural or caudal block, all entail problems: time consumed doing the block, potential technical difficulties with the block, time consumed waiting for onset, variability in degree of block produced, and problems in the recovery period.

Any degree of motor paralysis significantly prolongs recovery room time. While it is possible to send a patient from the recovery room back to the surgical ward with a small amount of residual block, the ambulatory patient cannot walk out to the car. The problem of postlumbar puncture headache is always a consideration and can significantly complicate the ambulatory surgical patient's course of recovery and early return to work. Perirectal field blocks, described in detail in another chapter, are employed for these reasons.

COMPLICATIONS

The most frequently reported complications in the Center at TMC are: nausea and vomiting (20 to 25 percent), headache, sore throat, and muscle pain. Shoulder pain is occasionally seen in the laparoscopic patients and is due to phrenic nerve irritation secondary to intraperitoneal insufflation.

In the series presented, 97 patients had problems necessitating transfer to a hospital. These problems or complications, with frequency, are listed below.

- Positive breast biopsies, 29 (One in 3 breast biopsies was positive.)
- Other positive biopsies, 8
- GYN complications secondary to laparoscopy (17), D and C (9), EIP (3), bleeding, bowel burns, viscus perforation
- Miscellaneous GYN: ectopic (1), post-repair (1), Skenes gland excision (1)
- GU complications, bleeding secondary to biopsy (10)
- Cryohemorrhoidectomy problems, 4
- Pacemaker complications, 1
- Attempts at skeletal pinning, 2
- A-V shunt revisions, 4
- T and A bleeding, 2
- Miscellaneous, 5

SUMMARY

The safety, economy and acceptability of the concept of the ambulatory surgical facility have been proved; its future depends upon the support it receives from us as physicians. The role of the anesthesiologist in the short-stay surgical facility is also well established.

REFERENCES

1. Nicole, J. H.: *The surgery of infancy.* Br. Med. J. 2:753, 1909.
2. Waters, R. M.: *The down-town anesthesia clinic.* Am. J. Surg. (Anesth. Suppl.) 33:71, 1919.
3. *Outpatient surgery: how and where should it be offered?* AMA News, June 6, 1977.
4. Davis, J. E.: *Day surgery: a viable alternative.* AORN J. 19:641–647, 1974.
5. Reed, W. A., and Ford, J. L.: *The SURGICENTER: an ambulatory surgical facility.* Clin. Obstet. Gynaecol. 17:217–230, 1974.
6. Eisenhammer, S.: *Internal anal sphincterotomy plus free dilation versus anal stretch with special criticism of the anal stretch procedure for hemorrhoids.* Dis. Colon Rectum 17:493–522, 1974.

2

THE CONCEPT OF THE SURGICENTER[R]

Wallace A. Reed, M.D.

The modern outpatient surgical unit is the brain child of anesthesiologists. Foremost in this field is Dr. Wallace Reed, cofounder of the Surgicenter[R] in Phoenix. Surgicenter[R] has served as the model for outpatient anesthesia and surgery, and is recognized as a highly efficient organization with an enviable safety record. In the following chapter, Dr. Reed discusses the concept of an outpatient surgical unit as embodied in the Surgicenter[R].

Burnell R. Brown, Jr.

The Surgicenter[R] concept is a new entity in the health care delivery system. The objective of the authors of the concept was to define a group of patients intermediate between those seen in the physician's office and those seen as inpatients in the surgical suite of a hospital, patients whose surgical care could be delivered safely in the outpatient environment.

The doctors believed in 1969, and have shown by implementation of the concept since then, that 20 to 40 percent of surgical procedures presently performed in hospitals can be safely handled on an outpatient basis. Almost any patient whose operation does not involve major intervention into cranial vault, thorax, or abdomen is a candidate for an outpatient surgical service. Not ideally suited for the outpatient environment are patients who may have postoperative pain unrelieved by oral analgesics, those whose operations are likely to be followed by postoperative bleeding, and those who have severe emotional objections to the idea or who live alone.

In developing the concept, it was found that it is safe to provide surgical care on an outpatient basis outside the administrative umbrella of the hospital and to a greater degree than had even been thought possible prior to 1970. Over 47,000 patients have been safely treated in the Surgicenter[R] since opening day, February 12, 1970. Not a single death has occurred in the six operating rooms of the Surgicenter[R]. The types of surgical problems treated have become progressively more complex, which is a testimony to surgeons' growing confidence in this innovation. Many other physicians have developed and are developing similar facilities in their own communities, as are many hospitals. Indications are that this intermediate level of surgical care represents a new entity in the health care delivery system.

The success derives from:

An ability to satisfy the unique needs of the patient requiring elective surgical care.

A willingness to meet the special demands of physicians and nurses working in the outpatient environment.

The public's increased interest in and knowledge of medical matters.

Careful methods of screening to assure that the patient's surgical problem is one that can be treated safely in the outpatient environment.

Improved anesthetic techniques, with great care employed in implementation.

The public's willingness to participate in the nursing of themselves and their families, thereby becoming "paramedics" of the best kind.

Growing acceptance by surgeons.

Wider acceptance and endorsement by companies offering health insurance benefits.

The patients' discovery that they are not treated like items of medical merchandise, but are respected as individuals in the surgical center environment.

Third party carriers, reluctant at the outset to recognize the freestanding surgical facilities as qualified providers, have become enthusiastic about the concept and are now promoting it widely. They have come to recognize the economic advantages of helping patients to stay "on their feet."

The Orkand Report* has been completed and has established that the cost of delivering this care is reduced in the freestanding outpatient surgical environment without loss of quality. It was found that:

There were no differences in complications.

There was little difference in the overall level of patient satisfaction, although the facilities physically separate from the hospital were somewhat more satisfactory in the minds of the patients.

The freestanding ambulatory surgical center rated higher than other settings in physician satisfaction.

The cost in the freestanding center was lower.

The quality of care as judged by outcome is as good as that found in the inpatient environment.

There were several features incorporated into the Surgicenter[R] concept that contributed to the cost containment discovered in the Orkand Study:

---

*The Orkand Report, performed under a 3-year $600,000 contract by the Orkand Corporation of Silver Spring, Maryland, was the first official HEW-funded study of the costs and impact of ambulatory surgery.

The facility was developed "from the ground up" for the purpose of serving the needs of the ambulatory patient exclusively.

Cost was reduced in construction of the facility by eliminating flammable anesthetics.

Simple laboratory tests reliably performed by nursing personnel were incorporated into the screening procedure.

Surgeons were permitted to read their patients' x-rays.

Referral to consulting radiologists was left to the discretion of the attending surgeons.

Twenty-four-hour laboratory and x-ray coverage were eliminated and reduced to the 6 AM to 6 PM ambulatory care schedule.

Cafeteria and laundry services were eliminated.

A total facility charge was set for each procedure, in order to set a ceiling such that quality care is provided within a reasonable budget. This provides incentive for health care to be delivered as economically as possible. Protection against under-treatment is assured by the surgeon's evaluation of the patient's outcome. Patients who feel they have been under-treated would not recommend the facility to friends, with the ultimate result that volume would diminish.

This level of care has its own novel medical environment. It is designed architecturally and conceptually to permit each member of personnel to function at his best. Surgeons and anesthesiologists practicing in the facility enjoy many attractive medical features. Studies have shown that patients are happier when sent home following a surgical procedure. Today's patients are more sophisticated in medical matters and are ready to assume a greater share of their own care.

Patients who are treated with honesty, respect, and skillful care don't take their doctors to court. This means that much of the medical cost related to "practicing defensively" can be eliminated in the Surgicenter[R] environment.*

---

*In its seven-year existence, only two suits have been brought against the Surgicenter[R]. In the first case, the plaintiff lost and was held responsible for court costs. In the second, the defense motion for a summary judgment with prejudice was granted; i.e., the plaintiff's complaint was judged to be without merit.

Personnel extend themselves to earn the trust of and establish rapport with patients by answering their questions and by giving good professional treatment while at the same time delivering that essential ingredient, compassionate care.

Finally, it is a part of the Surgicenter[R] concept to provide this care and this service under what has until recently been considered a questionable banner; i.e., as a proprietary entity. One of the objectives of the author has been to demonstrate how private capital can be attracted to the health care field. It is the author's opinion, based on studies from experiences in other countries, that the health care needed by the public cannot be supplied through government funding alone. The private sector must also contribute. The Surgicenter[R] is showing that this can be done. The fear expressed by some critics that there is danger of a few individuals reaping huge profits through the operation of a facility such as the Surgicenter[R] is not a valid one. It is invalid because there is such close surveillance through the Health Systems Agencies. In most instances an investor could obtain a better short-term return by purchasing tax-free municipal (or hospital) bonds. It is the author's intent to show that a proprietary entity can be just as public-spirited and often less hypocritical than facilities operating under the "nonprofit" label.

The Surgicenter[R], a contribution from the private medical sector, is a new entity in the health care delivery system. It serves the intermediate surgical patient and reduces cost while maintaining a high quality of care. It functions as an extension of the surgeon's office, thus permitting the elimination of many unnecessary laboratory and other screening tests. It has established an enviable safety record. The concept will thrive in proportion to the number of dedicated physicians who support its cause.

3

PREOPERATIVE ASSESSMENT OF THE PATIENT FOR OUTPATIENT ANESTHESIA

James B. Duckett, M.D.*

Never has the role of anesthesiologist as physician been more challenged than in outpatient evaluation. The dictum "there may be minor surgery but there are no minor anesthetics" is still warranted. Some are of the opinion that an accurate preanesthetic assessment is the most important part of anesthesia administration. The excellent safety records of anesthesiologist-manned facilities, such as the Surgicenter[R], indicate that training and experience in anesthesiology are the best preparation for patient assessment and the administration of anesthesia. This is not to discourage medical consultations. However, we do not ask the internist the best anesthetic technique for a particular patient—that is not his area of expertise. We ask him whether the patient is in optimal condition for the surgical-anesthetic experience. He arrives at this decision through his comprehensive review of the patient's history, physical examination, laboratory studies, and response to medications. Obviously, the approach to preoperative assessment will vary among anesthesiologists. This chapter provides the outline for such evaluation.

Burnell R. Brown, Jr.

*Deceased

Surgery on a patient who is admitted through a day surgery or an outpatient surgery unit is, by definition, minor surgery. However, there is no such thing as minor anesthesia. Therefore, the preoperative evaluation of a day surgery patient should be exceedingly accurate and painstakingly thorough. There may be a tendency in an outpatient surgery atmosphere to make a lot of assumptions; namely, that the patient is healthy and has been completely worked up by the surgeon, and that the anticipated surgery is indeed of short duration and of minor scope. Assumptions can be at best troublesome, and at worst, lethal.

The anesthesiologist must be certain that a complete medical history and physical examination have been performed, and any necessary laboratory tests done and the results reported, prior to administration of an anesthetic. A thorough knowledge of the patient's history, including previous anesthetic experience and physical and laboratory findings, enables the anesthesiologist to determine the patient's acceptability as an outpatient, and to determine the type of anesthetic to be used.[1] This knowledge also helps guard against serious problems arising during the course of the anesthesia and surgery.[2]

Several schemes have been suggested and are being used which enable the anesthesiologist to evaluate the patient prior to surgery. In some areas,[3, 4] the patient is seen by the anesthesiologist the day before the anticipated surgery, and necessary laboratory examinations are performed at this time. In this type of situation a history and physical examination have usually already been done in the surgeon's office or in the clinic, and the written record of the history and physical examination is either hand carried by the patient to the outpatient surgery unit, or the record is forwarded via intrahospital channels to the outpatient surgery unit. In other locations,[5, 6, 7] the patient is seen on the day of surgery, enough time being allowed for the anesthesiologist to evaluate and examine the patient and have basic laboratory tests run. In this sort of situation also, the history and physical examination will already have been performed in the surgeon's office within the preceding 1 or 2 weeks and forwarded to the outpatient surgery unit. Basic laboratory tests will have already been performed along with any other tests deemed necessary, and the results likewise forwarded to the outpatient unit. The reports of these examinations, as well as the patient's medical history and results of physical examination, are then available to the anesthesiologist for use during his preoperative evaluation.[1, 8]

Seeing the patient the day before surgery gives the anesthesiologist more time and a degree of flexibility not possible if he is to see the patient only shortly before surgery. It does entail another trip to the outpatient surgery clinic by the patient. Seeing the patient the day of surgery eliminates the extra trip by the patient, but requires a very efficient outpatient surgery facility with excellent communication among doctors, nurses, and administrative personnel.

When the patient is seen by the anesthesiologist, a preoperative medication, if desired, can be ordered. Most anesthesiologists dealing with outpatient anesthetics limit preoperative medications. In infants and children, an anticholinergic such as atropine or glycopyrrolate is usually ordered to be given intramuscularly shortly before surgery. Adults may receive either no preoperative medication or a mild sedative such as diazepam shortly before surgery. At Parkland Memorial Hospital, in Dallas, our routine procedure for adult outpatients who are to receive general or a regional anesthesia is 10 mg of diazepam, to be given orally with 30 ml of antacid, about 1 hour prior to surgery. Our experience favors the prophylactic use of a preoperative antacid. Oral diazepam is more effective than intramuscular administration of the drug. A more comprehensive review of premedication is found in Chapter 4 *(Role of Premedication in Outpatient Anesthesia).*

The selection of patients for outpatient surgery is made by the surgeon. Epstein[9] has listed some of the factors that should be considered in deciding whether or not a patient should have outpatient surgery:

Simplicity of the procedure, which should be less than 90 minutes in length, have minimal anticipated bleeding and minimal physiologic derangements.
Procedure's reliably low incidence of postoperative complications.
General good health of the patient.
Reliability of the patient, if an adult.
The patient's motivation to have the surgery.
Cooperation of the surgeon.

Surgical procedures should be chosen that are not expected to exceed 90 minutes. This involves a total anesthetic time of 100 to 130 minutes, depending on the institution, surgeon, surgery, and the anesthesiologist. I feel that a total anesthetic time of greater than 2 hours is excessive for an outpatient as it leads to prolonged recovery time and increased morbidity, not only the day of surgery but also the next day.

Total surgical and anesthesia time are not the only considerations. Outpatient surgery should be limited to procedures with little bleeding and minimal physiologic derangements.[10] A laparoscopic tubal "ligation" or fulguration is a case for consideration. This procedure involves intubation of the trachea, controlled ventilation, and profound relaxation for a short time. The patient must be awake, breathing spontaneously, and the trachea extubated, all in as short a time as possible. In this type of procedure , which usually lasts only 10 to 20 minutes, the time spent in the recovery room and in the outpatient area before discharge often totals 4 to 6 hours. This is a good illustration of the fact that a short operative procedure does not necessarily require a short recovery period.

Surgical procedures should be simple and should entail a predictably low rate of postoperative complications. Operations known to have a moderate incidence of postoperative problems or morbidity, even if the procedure is short, should not be done on an outpatient basis. A tonsillectomy and adenoidectomy is considered by some not to be suitable for outpatient surgery because of the relatively high risk of postoperative bleeding.

Subjects for outpatient surgery should be generally healthy, usually ASA Class I.[1, 7, 10] Patients with well controlled systemic disease (e.g. those in ASA Class II) are often good candidates for outpatient surgery. The anesthesiologist's preoperative evaluation is necessary to ascertain the status of the patient's health, and to enable the anesthesiologist to order any required laboratory tests as indicated by the patient's medications.

The primary considerations in the suitability of a patient for outpatient surgery are the patient's individualized needs, the contemplated surgery and anesthetic, and the patient's physical and psychological status. Excellent communication and understanding between the surgeon and the anesthesiologist is mandatory. If there is any question of the patient's fitness for outpatient surgery, the surgeon and the anesthesiologist should discuss the case and decide whether or not the patient might be better managed as an inpatient. Patients with diabetes mellitus or hypertension that is not well controlled are examples of patients who might be admitted to the hospital or have surgery postponed while the systemic disease is brought under better control.

The patient should be well motivated to have his surgery done on an outpatient basis. The person who has been pushed into outpatient surgery by an enthusiastic surgeon, friend, or relative but is himself very frightened makes a poor candidate indeed. This person is far more likely to require overnight admission to a hospital for many reasons, some physiologic, some psychologic. In our experience at Parkland Memorial Hospital, in our recently established Day Surgery Unit, we have had an inpatient admission rate, from September 1, 1976, to September 1, 1977, of 29 out of 902 outpatients. Of these 29 patients, 5 were admitted solely at their own request.

As the surgeon is the initiator of the outpatient surgical experience, he usually provides the patient with specific written instructions. If the surgeon does not perform this duty, the patient should receive instructions from the outpatient surgery unit personnel. It is imperative that the patient receive, read, understand, and agree to these instructions. The instructions should include the entire schedule for the patient, i.e., when and where to appear for preoperative anesthesia evaluation, for admission procedures, and for laboratory tests, and when and where to appear for surgery. The surgeon or outpatient unit personnel must be sure that the directions are understood, emphasize the importance of following them exactly, and elicit the patient's promise to do so. If the patient is unable to understand the instructions or is unwilling or unable to follow them, he is not a candidate for outpatient surgery.

The following specific points must be understood and adhered to by the patient.

1. The patient should not take any food or drink after the midnight before surgery. Brushing of teeth or rinsing of the mouth is acceptable if the patient understands that he should not swallow anything. Most patients will readily follow instructions if they understand the importance of being NPO prior to administration of an anesthetic.

2. The patient must agree to report to the surgeon or the anesthesiologist any change in physical condition (cold, fever, sore throat, etc.). Patients tend to want to proceed with scheduled surgery in spite of any newly developed "sniffles", especially after spending parts of at least 2 or 3 days arranging for the operation. If the potential danger of a general anesthetic in face of a recent URI or fever is understood, most patients will agree to reschedule the procedure.

3. It must be understood that discharge will not be made in the absence of a responsible adult. Explanation of the known[9-15] inability to drive a car or function normally for 12 to 24 hours following a general, regional or local (with sedation) anesthetic is usually sufficient to convince even skeptical patients of the need for assistance in getting home, whether by car or taxi.

4. The patient must agree to refrain for 24 hours from alcoholic beverages or any medication not prescribed or acknowledged by the surgeon and anesthesiologist.

5. The patient must agree to refrain for 24 hours from making important decisions and from operating complicated machinery. (What constitutes "complicated machinery" should be evaluated for each case.)

6. The patient should submit in writing names and telephone numbers of those to contact, or where to come, should a complication develop after the patient has gone home. If the patient lives out of town, an overnight stay near the hospital on the night following surgery is highly recommended.

The form instructing the patient in these points should be read and signed by the patient during the admitting process and made part of his record. This is to insure as well as possible that the patient gives informed consent to the rather special procedures involved in outpatient surgery.[7]

A history, physical examination, blood count, and urinalysis are required of any patient having a regional or general anesthetic. Institutions vary in their timing regulations. For some institutions, 1 or 2 weeks prior to surgery is adequate for a history and physical exam, while other institutions' pre-admission procedures require that all of the work-up be done within 24 hours of the scheduled surgery. A history and physical examination done a few days before surgery may necessitate an extra trip to the surgeon's office or to the hospital, but the inconvenience is far outweighed by the improved screening of patients and the reduced incidence of cancelled cases on the day of surgery. Not only is patient safety improved, but operative scheduling and efficiency are enhanced. Basic laboratory tests should be run 1 to 10 days prior to surgery, depending on the institutional policy. Extra laboratory tests, as indicated by the patient's history, age, physical exam, or medications, may be obtained as needed, provided a sufficient interval is available to permit the interpretation of these examinations before the scheduled surgery. Obviously, the time interval should be long enough so that last minute surgery cancellations are avoided. The best example that I know of is the determination of serum potassium of patients who are taking diuretics, especially thiazide diuretics.

The anesthesiologist should always reserve the right to decide whether the patient is a physical and psychological candidate for outpatient anesthesia.[16] The anesthesiologist should also be alert to ambitious surgery scheduled by a zealous surgeon who feels that *he* can perform *this* particular operation on *this* particular patient in an "acceptable" amount of time, with an "acceptable" morbidity and blood loss. Referring again to our experience over the last year at Parkland Memorial Hospital, of the 29 (out of 902) patients admitted following an outpatient surgical procedure, 15 were admitted for surgical reasons such as surgery more extensive than was anticipated or need for more postoperative care and observation than was anticipated. Of the remaining patients of the group of 29, 4 had planned to be admitted (patients having tonsillectomy and adenoidectomy or from out of town), 2 were operated on too late in the day to return to our Day Surgery Unit for discharge, and 3 were admitted for anesthesia-related problems such as nausea and vomiting, and prolonged intubation. One patient was too sleepy to go home following a late-scheduled and prolonged x-ray examination.

Any questions in the anesthesiologist's mind should be immediately aired with the surgeon, and a conclusion reached. Good communication between the surgeon and the anesthesiologist is crucial if patient safety and efficient utilization of the facilities are to be achieved. Only through open and honest discussion between these two physicians can these interests be well served. Unacceptable procedures must never be attempted, and the patient's safety must never be compromised. Questionable risks should be identified before an anesthetic is administered, and "short cuts" should be avoided.

I do not propose that the anesthesiologist should be a "watch dog," but that he should be a member of the team, with a voice in the patient's treatment. The anesthesiologist is involved with the case as a consulting physician who, above all else, has the patient's safety in mind.

REFERENCES

1. Schmidt, K. F.: *Evaluation of candidates for outpatient anesthesia and surgery.* Int. Anesth. Clin. 14:9–13, 1976.
2. Ogg, T. W.: *Assessment of pre-operative cases.* Br. Med. J. 1:82–83, 1976.
3. Ahlgren, E. W., Bennett, E. J., and Stephen, C. R.: *Outpatient pediatric anesthesiology—a case series.* Anesth. Analg. (Cleve) 50:402–408, 1971.
4. Patterson, J. F., Bechtoldt, A. A., and Levin, K. J.: *Ambulatory surgery in a university setting.* JAMA 235:266–268, 1976.
5. Levy, M. L., and Coakley, C. S.: *Organization and experience with outpatient anesthesia in a large university hospital.* Int. Anesth. Clin. 14:131–142, 1976.
6. *Surgicenters—new idea for one day surgery.* Resident and Staff Physician, April, 1973.
7. Thompson, G. E., Remington, J. M., Millman, B. S., et al.: *Experiences with outpatient anesthesia.* Anesth. Analg. (Cleve) 52:881–887, 1973.
8. Janis, K. M., and Downs, J. B.: *The anesthesia screening clinic—Letters to the Editor.* JAMA 223:692, 1973.
9. Epstein, B. S.: *Outpatient anesthesia.* ASA Refresher Courses in Anesthesiology 2:81–96, 1974.
10. Jones, C. W.: *Anesthesia for outpatient surgery.* J. Natl. Med. Assoc. 66:411–415, 1974.
11. Baird, E. S., and Harley, D. M.: *Delayed recovery from a sedative: correlation of the plasma levels of diazepam with clinical effects after oral and intravenous administration.* Br. J. Anaesth. 44:803–807, 1972.
12. Doenicke, A., Kugler, J., and Laub, M.: *Evaluation of recovery and "street fitness" by EEG and psychodiagnostic tests after anesthesia.* Can. Anaesth. Soc. J. 14:567–583, 1967.
13. Fahy, A., and Marshal, M.: *Postanesthetic morbidity in outpatients.* Br. J. Anaesth. 41:433–438, 1969.
14. Korttila, K.: *Minor outpatient anesthesia and driving.* Mod. Probl. Pharmacopsychiatry 11:91–98, 1976.

15. Newman, M. G., Trieger, N., and Miller, J. C.: *Measuring recovery from anesthesia—a simple test.* Anesth. Analg. (Cleve) 48:136–140, 1969.
16. Coakley, C. S., and Levey, M. L.: *Anesthesia for ambulatory surgery.* J. Ark. Med. Soc. 68:101–104, 1971.

4

ROLE OF PREMEDICATION IN OUTPATIENT ANESTHESIA

M. Lawrence Cobb, M.D., and
C. Ronald Stephen, M.D.

There is general consensus that premedication has no role in outpatient anesthesia. Since the objective is to have a patient as awake and reactive as possible, it follows logically that "fixed" drugs used as premedicants defeat this purpose. Yet, as in all cases, there are exceptions and debates; the use of anticholinergics is an example. Drs. Cobb and Stephen explore this controversial issue. Although no absolute indications are put forth, their information should afford the practicing anesthesiologist a base on which to synthesize his own approach to the problem.

Burnell R. Brown, Jr.

Some might say that preanesthetic medication has no role in outpatient anesthesia. Such a statement is justified if the primary aim of outpatient anesthesia is simply the patient's rapid return to normal functioning.[14] The omission of premedication may not be in keeping with the best patient care, however, even though in recent papers the topic is ignored or condemned.[10, 14] It would be timely to review some of the reasons that premedication has become so deeply rooted in the management of patients about to be anesthetized, and then determine whether omission would be beneficial or harmful to the outpatient.

Because of physiologic variations between adults and children, particularly with respect to biotransformation of drugs and relative dominance of the sympathetic vs parasympathetic nervous system[5], it is wise to consider the desirability of outpatient premedication in each of these two age groups.

PEDIATRIC PATIENTS

In a recently published article, R. M. Smith wrote, "We have not yet found either a suitable tranquilizing agent to help children tolerate hospitalization or a satisfactory method of preanesthetic sedation. Instead, we continue to inject illogical doses of unpredictable agents."[12]

An ideal premedicant for these patients is given orally, is rapidly absorbed, and has a predictable onset and a relatively short duration of action (2 to 3 hours). It produces a tranquil, sleepy (but arousable) child cooperative during induction of anesthesia. Ideally, vagal mediated bradycardia is prevented during anesthesia, as are sialorrhea and bronchorrhea, but an uncomfortably dry mouth is not present. Postoperative analgesia is present without respiratory, cardiovascular, or central nervous system depression. Nausea and vomiting are suppressed in the pre- and postoperative periods. Obviously, such an ideal drug has not been found.

Any discussion of premedication for the pediatric outpatient must take into account several peculiarities inherent in the outpatient situation. Duration of action of any drug must be a prime consideration because the child will return home within 2 or 3 hours after the anesthesia and surgery. The pediatric age group most often coming to the operating room is below the age of self-care. Therefore, drug prescription must take into consideration the effects of those drugs on the care of that child by the parent(s) after the child leaves the hospital. In addition, one must think about the kind of surgery to be performed and the anticipated severity of postoperative pain. Finally, compatibility between the planned anesthetic management and premedicant drugs deserves careful thought.

Several reviews of pediatric outpatient anesthesia have been published in the last 6 years.[1, 4, 13] Either a belladonna drug[1, 13] preceding an inhalation induction of anesthesia, oral diazepam in the particularly apprehensive child,[1] or no premedication[1, 4] have been used, all with success.

When one considers premedicant drugs, three basic groups emerge: anticholinergic drugs, sedatives and tranquilizers, and narcotics. These groups will be discussed separately, and the pros and cons of each group considered, as they apply to the pediatric outpatient.

Anticholinergics

Many anesthesiologists strongly believe that every pediatric patient should receive a parenterally administered anticholinergic drug prior to a general anesthetic. However, recent reports[7, 9] indicate that some authors question the routine use of this group of drugs, at least in adults. Some 15 years ago, Eger concluded a review article on anticholinergics with the statement, "The time has come when the use of the belladonna drugs should be tailored to circumstance and not given by rote."[5] It is worth remembering that the routine use of parasympatholytics did have a firm rationale when irritant anesthetic vapors were commonly employed. The copious upper airway and bronchial secretions resulted in airway obstruction, prolonged induction, and sometimes laryngospasm. However, the inhalation agents of today, primarily halothane and enflurane, do not stimulate these secretions.

To produce reliable antisialagogue effects, atropine and scopolamine are given parenterally, with specific preanesthetic timing.[15] There is much made of the fact that anesthesia and operation on an outpatient basis have as a major advantage minimal psychologic trauma to the child. Further, great efforts are made to manage the induction phase so that further emotional trauma is not inflicted. Few would argue these goals, yet some would not hesitate to have a third party give the child a painful injection just prior to separation from the parents. One wonders whether such an injection does not produce sufficient anxiety in the child to offset the subsequent careful atraumatic induction. There is no doubt that many children have a real aversion to needles. This is not to say that a needed injection should not be given, but to question whether the benefit is really worth the effect on the child; in other words, to suggest that one assess the benefit to risk ratio. One rarely finds an adult who looks forward to an injection, particularly one of questionable value that produces a dry mouth and no relief from either pain or apprehension. A child cannot be expected to understand or accept such an injection with greater ease than would an adult.

In several specific situations, however, premedication with an antisialagogue is important. If either intravenous or intramuscular ketamine is to be used (e.g. for outpatient radiation therapy), then atropine should be given intramuscularly 15 to 45 minutes prior to ketamine. If awake tracheal intubation is anticipated in an outpatient infant—our youngest pediatric outpatient was 5 days old—atropine is useful in reducing the outpouring of secretions secondary to awake laryngoscopy. Finally, if a peroral endoscopic procedure is to be performed, secretions will be much less a problem to the surgeon if a belladonna drug has been administered.

Other reasons for administering an anticholinergic agent exist. One is for prevention of undesirable vagal reflexes, particularly bradycardia. If succinylcholine is to be injected intravenously to facilitate endotracheal intubation, atropine can be mixed with the succinylcholine in the same syringe to effectively prevent bradycardia. If a child is to have an eye procedure during which traction may be placed on the extraocular muscles, atropine is certainly appropriate. Atropine given intravenously in a dose of 0.02 mg per kg during an inhalation or intravenous induction of anesthesia is probably far more effective in preventing the oculocardiac reflex than when given as a preoperative medication by the intramuscular route.

Another frequently discussed use of one of the newer anticholinergic compounds, glycopyrrolate, is a reduction of the volume and acidity of gastric secretions. However, an oral pediatric dose form of this drug is neither available nor has it been proven effective. A study of the value of parenteral glycopyrrolate in pediatric patients[11] claimed a reduction in gastric volume and acidity, but an unreliable means of determining the volume of gastric contents was used. Further, the clinical importance and risk of the presence of a small volume of liquid in the stomach of a healthy child scheduled for a short elective procedure is unknown. Provided that the airway is properly cared for, the difference between 4 ml and 20 ml of fluid in the stomach may be academic. In a fasting child without gastrointestinal tract pathology, regurgitation and aspiration should not occur unless uncorrected airway obstruction develops. An unanswered question is whether the uncomfortable side effect of dry mouth outweighs the rare phenomenon of vomitus aspiration. More to the point is the question of gastric acidity. Careful study of an oral preparation appears to be indicated to answer this complex issue of volume and total acidity, as well as the issue of risk/benefit ratio.

Barbiturates, Hypnotics, and Tranquilizers

Many hypnotic and/or anxiety-relieving drugs have been proposed for premedication in the pediatric patient. All of these drugs appear to share one or both of the following shortcomings: their effects are not satisfactorily predictable; and/or they have a duration of action incompatible with a rapid recovery of awareness and appropriate responsiveness to various stimuli, particularly pain.

Barbiturates have long been used to sedate children preoperatively, though not without several problems. One of these is the paradoxical excitement occasionally seen following the administration of barbiturates either parenterally or orally. Such reactions probably indicate suboptimal dosage. However, to insure optimal dose in all patients results in prolonged sedation in many. A further problem is the "emergence delirium" all too commonly seen postoperatively in patients who are having pain and who have received a barbiturate for premedication.

The useful hypnotics and tranquilizers include oral triclofos or chloral hydrate (both are metabolized to the same effective compound, trichlorethanol), oral diazepam, parenteral hydroxyzine, and parenteral droperidol. Of these compounds, orally administered diazepam[3, 13] and triclofos[3] would seem to have advantages. However, information related to the time required for postanesthetic recovery following administration of these drugs in children is absent. Droperidol, in addition to requiring an injection, produces many desirable effects preoperatively. Unfortunately, in our experience it prolongs recovery to an unacceptable extent. Hydroxyzine as a sole premedicant has few proponents, possibly because of the pain it produces given intramuscularly.

Narcotics

Unless narcotics are administered preoperatively as an integral part of the intraoperative anesthetic management, there is little rationale for use. Certainly, the additive respiratory depressant effects of an analgesic dose of a narcotic plus adequate depth of a potent inhalation agent mitigate against physiologic spontaneous ventilation during anesthesia. The agent most frequently used for pediatric outpatient anesthesia is halothane. Premedication with a narcotic would almost force tracheal intubation and/or controlled ventilation for a relatively brief procedure that otherwise could be performed with spontaneous ventilation.

In addition, the duration of action of the commonly used narcotics, except for fentanyl, results in delayed emergency and delayed recovery. As a result, the time interval from the beginning of the recovery period until the child can safely be discharged from the outpatient unit, able to tolerate liquids, void, and ambulate, may well be 4 to 6 hours rather than 1 to 2 hours. This is not to say that we oppose either tracheal intubation or pain relief. In fact, approximately 50 percent of our pediatric outpatients require an endotracheal tube. If a patient develops significant discomfort postoperatively, fentanyl is administered intramuscularly. Such medication is occasionally needed in the older child who has had a circumcision, orchiopexy, umbilical herniorrhaphy, or cystoscopy.

Psychologic Premedication

The concept of adequate psychologic preparation of a child for an operative procedure is not new.[8] Although this approach requires considerable time and the ability to talk to a child on his/her own level, the effort can be most rewarding. Interviews have been conducted with children who have had an inhalation induction for a minor surgical procedure such as that currently done on an outpatient basis.[2] The findings indicate that, regardless of pharmacologic premedication, the child's own ability to cope with stress was a major factor in his response to the anesthetic experience. It is in this sphere that the sensitive anesthesiologist who participates in helping the child prepare for an anesthetic can usually contribute far more by spending time with the child preoperatively than he can by prescribing drugs. Since the child is also very much attuned to parental anxieties about anesthesia and operation, it is also vital to address the parents' fears. This can be accomplished by providing factual information to the parents and by being an "active listener" genuinely open to their expressed anxieties. One must also remember that personnel other than the anesthesiologist can help in the emotional preparation of the child and parents. Their abilities to impart information to parents and children can contribute much to the overall preparation of the child for anesthesia and operation.

"What We Do"

In our pediatric outpatient anesthetic preparation, premedicant drugs are administered rarely.

All patients come to the short stay unit on the afternoon prior to the day of operation. During this visit both parents and child are oriented to the unit, intercurrent illness is ruled out, and plans for the anesthetic are discussed with the patient and parents.

The nurses in the short stay unit begin by a brief explanation to the parent(s) and child of the functioning of the unit. The child and parent(s) are then shown an album of photographs of a child in various stages of a short stay admission. Events such as the physical examination, riding on a stretcher to the operating room, lying on the operating room table, being anesthetized via an inhalation induction, awakening in the recovery room, and returning to the unit and awaiting parents are depicted. The child is encouraged to ask questions that the nurses attempt to answer as forthrightly as possible. Great effort is made to tell the child the truth about the events of the operative day. Next, a history and physical examination are completed by the surgeon, and the child and parent(s) are interviewed by the anesthesiologist. The anesthetic-related events are discussed again with the child and family, with an effort to make the child feel as much a participant in the discussion as possible. Obviously, it is important to gear the level of conversation to the age of the child. A brochure prepared by the St. Louis Children's Hospital is given to the parents. It reinforces information about when to make the child NPO and what time to report to the short stay unit the next day, and provides general information pertinent to the outpatient unit.

When the patient comes to the operating room the next day, a nurse whom the child met the previous day accompanies the patient. This nurse stays with the child, usually holding his hand until induction of anesthesia is completed. This type of preparation has been a most satisfactory form of "premedication" in our pediatric outpatients. When weighed against the undesirable side effects of the available alternatives, we judge it to be preferable to any currently available premedicant drugs or combinations thereof. Nevertheless, we anxiously await the availability of that elusive "ideal" premedicant drug which would eliminate unpleasantness for the child and leave only happy memories of the outpatient experience.

ADULT PATIENTS

The primary reasons for prescribing premedication have often been stated: 1) to alleviate preoperative pain; 2) to allay fear and apprehension; 3) to contribute to the management of the anesthetic; and 4) to reduce the incidence of secretions and vagal activity during anesthesia. To what extent are these reasons applicable to the outpatient having surgery? The situation in the United States and Canada is probably different from that in the United Kingdom, in that overseas such operations as herniorrhaphy and stripping of varicose veins are routinely performed on adults on an outpatient basis, whereas such procedures are a rare phenomenon in North America. The following remarks will be limited to experiences in the United States.

Except for occasional instances when fractures are to be treated on an outpatient basis, outpatients usually do not suffer pain preoperatively and there is, therefore, no indication to prescribe a pain-relieving drug, e.g., a narcotic, prior to inducing anesthesia. Moreover, there are substantial reasons for not prescribing narcotic premedication, for these drugs induce nausea in up to 25 percent of people and produce a degree of peripheral vasodilation which can result in orthostatic hypotension. This latter can compound the light-headedness and dizziness which patients often complain of when they first sit up or begin to walk in the recovery period. An exception to the rule may be the narcotic addict, in whom a titrated dose of a narcotic given intravenously just prior to induction of anesthesia is often physiologically beneficial.

Almost all adult patients approach an anesthetic and surgical experience with some degree of fear and apprehension. Most often, the anxiety is due to the unknown nature of what is to happen, but it may be fear of bodily harm, of not waking up, of feeling pain during the operation, and so on. Franklin Roosevelt in the dark days of the Second World War said, "We have nothing to fear but fear itself." And so in the outpatient, in whom as a general principle one wishes to avoid pharmacologic preanesthetic medication, the importance of psychologic premedication becomes paramount. Such means of alleviating fright call upon the exercise of the best traits of the anesthesiologist in his contact with the patient preoperatively. Perhaps "communication" best describes the process. There must be liaison and rapport established between the anesthesiologist and the patient if alarm and trepidation are to be reduced. There must be an interest shown in the social, as well as the physical, background of the patient. A careful explanation of what is going to happen, provided with an air of quiet confidence, will make known to the patient what was unknown. No conversation should end without the patient being asked if he/she has any questions. Ideally, one ends with the equivalent of a fully informed consent.

Sedative and tranquilizer drugs are frequently prescribed to inpatients to help alleviate preoperative distress. Is there any role for such drugs in the outpatient? If the communication prior to anesthesia has been adequate, probably not. However, if the patient has been receiving a tranquilizer regularly (and many today do so), or if the fear of the forthcoming procedure has not been eradicated despite full communication, such premedication may be considered. Diazepam 5 to 10 mg orally with a sip of water 1 to 2 hours before the operation may be indicated in such patients. In the young or middle-aged patient without concurrent hepatic disease, the sedative effects should be minimal in the recovery period.

With the relatively short duration of outpatient surgery and with the potent anesthetic drugs available, there is little need for premedication. The anesthesiologist can better estimate the required doses of anesthetic drugs if he does not have to take into account previously administered compounds, particularly narcotics.

Finally, one must consider the potential advantages or drawbacks of the preanesthetic administration of anticholinergic drugs. With present-day anesthetics, except for ketamine, the problem of inducing significant secretions is not significant, so there is no reason to prescribe anticholinergics on this account. However, consideration must be given to the potential for increased vagal tone developing during the anesthetic, promoted by drugs such as halothane or induced by anesthetic or surgical manipulation. To say that a drug, such as atropine, should be prescribed routinely is probably neither reasonable nor logical, as no two patients can be considered to be similar for such a requirement. In any given patient, as far as the conduction system of the heart is concerned, a certain balance exists between the influence of the sympathetic and parasympathetic nervous systems, and this influence can change from moment to moment. If a patient is under stress, in spite of all one's efforts, as may happen just before induction of anesthesia without premedication, sympathetic tone may be dominant, the pulse rate may be 80 to 90 per minute, and there is obviously no need for an anticholinergic drug. On the other hand, if the patient is phlegmatic, and fear has been abolished, the pulse rate may be 50 to 60 per minute. Under these circumstances, particularly if a sympatholytic drug such as halothane is to be administered, a degree of vagal blockade may be indicated. This is accomplished by administering atropine 0.3 to 0.5 mg intravenously to the patient 3 to 4 minutes prior to induction of anesthesia.

Some anesthesiologists believe that if a potent inhalation anesthetic such as halothane is to be administered, it should always be preceded by administration of atropine in order to avoid significant bradycardia or ventricular arrhythmias. In a recent study[6] it was demonstrated that in adults undergoing minor surgery with N_2O, O_2 and halothane without tracheal intubation, the incidence of arrhythmias in a control group was no higher than in patients who received atropine 0.1 mg per 10 kg intravenously 5 minutes prior to induction.

During the course of anesthesia and surgery, circumstances may develop which are associated with a significant bradycardia, a fall in blood pressure, and at times the development of ventricular arrhythmias, all signs of a potent vagal reaction. The obvious treatment is atropine intravenously, which may, however, during the transitional 2- or 3-minute period while autonomic balance is being restored, be associated with multiple bizarre and frightening arrhythmias. Such arrhythmias can be of concern, although they are almost invariably self-limited. This type of reaction can be avoided if one can predict this sequence of events, either by recognizing a relative increase in vagal tone prior to anesthesia, or by anticipating a potential surgical stimulus during the operation. If one is in doubt about the autonomic cardiac status of the patient before induction of anesthesia, it is probably wise to administer atropine intravenously before proceeding. By employing this prophylactic measure, one may avoid undesirable vagal reactions during the procedure and prevent additional upsets in cardiac rhythm which may develop if therapy is administered after the fact.

REFERENCES

1. Ahlgren, E. W., Bennett, E. J., and Stephen, C. R.: *Outpatient pediatric anesthesiology: a case series.* Anesth. Analg. (Cleve) 50:402–408, 1971.
2. Booth, A., and Galdston, R.: *The child's loss of consciousness: a psychiatric view of pediatric anesthesia.* Pediatrics 50:252–263, 1972.
3. Boyd, J. B., and Manford, M. L. M.: *Premedication in children.* Br. J. Anaesth. 45:501–506, 1973.
4. Cloud, D. T., Reed, W. A., Ford, J. L., et al.: *The Surgicenter: a fresh concept in outpatient pediatric surgery.* J. Pediatr. Surg. 7:206–212, 1972.
5. Eger, E. I., II: *Atropine, scopolamine, and related compounds.* Anesthesiology 23:365–383, 1962.
6. Eikard, B., and Anderson, J. R.: *Arrhythmias during halothane anaesthesia II: the influence of atropine.* Acta Anaesth. Scand. 21:245, 1977.

7. Famewo, C. E.: *A re-evaluation of anticholinergic premedication.* Can. Anaesth. Soc. J. 24:39–41, 1977.
8. Jackson, K.: *Psychologic preparation as a method of reducing the emotional trauma of anesthesia in children.* Anesthesiology 12:293–300, 1951.
9. Leighton, K. M., and Sanders, H. D.: *Anticholinergic premedication.* Can. Anaesth. Soc. J. 23:563–566, 1976.
10. Ogg, T. W.: *An assessment of postoperative outpatient cases.* Br. Med. J. 4:573, December 9, 1972.
11. Salem, M. R., Wong, A. Y., Mani, M., et al.: *Premedicant drugs and gastric juice pH and volume in pediatric patients.* Anesthesiology 44:216–219, 1976.
12. Smith, R. M.: *The pediatric anesthetist, 1950–1975.* Anesthesiology 43:144–155, 1975.
13. Steward, D. J.: *Outpatient pediatric anesthesia.* Anesthesiology 43:268–276, 1975.
14. Urbach, G. M., and Edelist, G.: *An evaluation of the anaesthetic techniques used in an outpatient unit.* Can. Anaesth. Soc. J. 24:401, May, 1977.

5

NITROUS-NARCOTIC-RELAXANT ANESTHESIA VS. VOLATILE ANESTHESIA IN THE ADULT SURGICAL OUTPATIENT

Casey Blitt, M.D.

What is the proper general anesthetic sequence to be administered for ambulatory surgery? Dr. Blitt reviews the advantages and disadvantages of inhaled versus intravenous anesthesia. The onus of selection of the appropriate technique is still upon the anesthesiologist after his assessment of the patient's physical and mental status, the anticipated surgery, and the skill of the surgeon.

Burnell R. Brown, Jr.

To clarify this discussion, I will first define nitrous-narcotic-relaxant anesthesia vs. volatile anesthetics. In the outpatient setting most general anesthetics (in adults) begin with an intravenous injection of an ultra-short-acting barbiturate (thiopental, thiamylal, methohexital). Most outpatients do not receive preanesthetic medication. Following barbiturate induction, nitrous oxide is administered in various concentrations. It is after this point in the anesthetic sequence that the two methods of administering anesthesia differ. What are the differences? The volatile anesthetics commonly employed are halothane, enflurane, and at times methoxyflurane. A nitrous-narcotic-relaxant technique consists of intravenous drugs added to 60 to 70 percent inspired nitrous oxide to obtain an "adequate" depth of anesthesia by producing sedation/hypnosis (sleep), amnesia, analgesia, and/or muscle relaxation. The volatile anesthetic agents are used by themselves (with or without nitrous oxide) to produce complete anesthesia and are used infrequently as sole anesthetic agents. Intravenous drugs include Innovar[R], three narcotics (morphine, meperidine, fentanyl), and ultra-short-acting barbiturates, all with or without neuromuscular blockers of the depolarizing or nondepolarizing type. These drugs are used in combination with nitrous oxide to produce a satisfactory (complete) anesthetic. The volatile anesthetic agents are frequently used in combination with neuromuscular blocking agents in outpatient anesthesia. The concept can be represented by a pyramid with nitrous oxide in the center and analgesia, muscle relaxation, sedation/sleep, and amnesia at the corners.

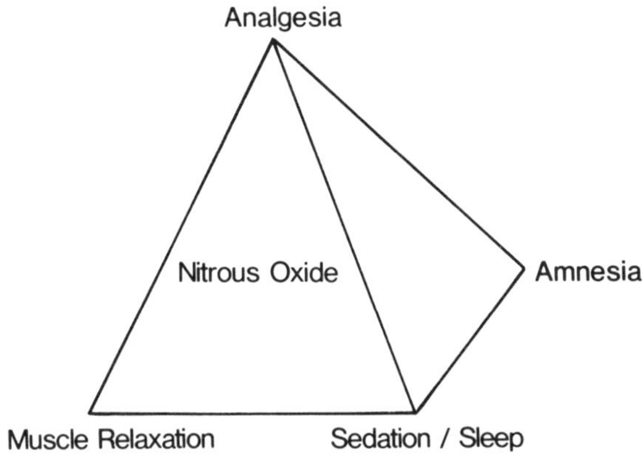

Thus, with nitrous oxide as an anesthetic base we provide the remaining components of a general anesthetic by either inhalation or by intravenous injection. What are the advantages and the disadvantages of these two types of anesthetics (inhaled vs. injected)? I will discuss the advantages and disadvantages in the following areas:

Retrievability and control of the anesthetic
Cost
Toxicity
Cardiovascular effects
Respiratory effects
Muscle relaxation and neuromuscular blocking agents
Recovery room
Awareness during anesthesia
Skill limitations and inherent limitations of technique
Miscellaneous

RETRIEVABILITY AND CONTROL

The inhaled agents are more easily eliminated from the body than are fixed agents. Once a fixed agent is administered it must be biotransformed by the liver and/or excreted via the kidney. The lung enables the volatile inhaled agents to be easily administered and easily excreted. Halothane and enflurane, with low blood gas solubility and high volatility, can be rapidly administered and eliminated. Because of low volatility and high blood gas solubility, methoxyflurane is difficult to administer for short procedures and the effects are prolonged. Despite the fact that there is a specific antagonist for narcotics (with the possible exception of fentanyl), care must be taken in administering narcotics and antagonists that the antagonist will outlast the duration of action of the narcotic. This can usually be accomplished by administering the naloxone intramuscularly as well as intravenously. If neuromuscular blocking agents have been used, recovery from these drugs either by natural dissipation of action or pharmacological antagonism must be verified, preferably by testing with a peripheral nerve stimulator.

Anesthetic depth is easily controlled with the inhaled agents because the inspired concentration of an inhalation agent is usually a reasonable guide to depth of anesthesia. Utilizing the concept of MAC (minimum alveolar concentration), the 95 percent confidence limit (1.25 MAC) of the concentration necessary to anesthetize a given patient is easily determined. Depth of anesthesia is easily controlled and it is easy to either withdraw or increase the anesthetic effect.

Some of the changes in vital signs occurring during anesthesia are more useful in determining anesthetic depth with inhaled than with injected agents. Classically blood pressure, respiratory rate and pattern, heart rate, and eye signs are used by anesthesiologists to gauge depth of anesthesia. Pulse rate and blood pressure, although reasonably good indicators of depth of anesthesia with volatile agents, are not very useful in nitrous-narcotic-relaxant anesthesia. Indeed, in healthy adult patients one often has a problem controlling hypertension which may develop in patients anesthetized with this technique. Respiratory rate and pattern are of value in both techniques but will be lost or markedly attenuated if neuromuscular blockers are employed. Eye signs are considerably more valuable in gauging depth of anesthesia with inhalation agents. Tearing, however, is valuable in both techniques for detecting light levels of anesthesia.

COST

The same anesthetic equipment (monitoring devices, etc.) is used to administer all general anesthetics. Thus certain volatile agents are more expensive than injected agents. Obviously, marked cost reductions can be effected by reducing gas flow. If gas flow is reduced markedly it is necessary to continuously monitor the concentration of oxygen in the exhalation limb of the anesthetic circuit. Estimating that 1 ml of liquid volatile agent vaporizes to approximately 200 ml of vapor, 20 ml of liquid enflurane are required to administer 2 percent inspired enflurane for 1 hour with a 3 L total flow and 40 ml using a 6 L total flow. With halothane (1 percent) the amount of liquid consumed is roughly $^{1}/_{3}$ of enflurane at flows of $2^{1}/_{2}$ and 5 L, respectively. A 125 ml bottle of enflurane costs $24.00, halothane, $11.00 (average wholesale price). The injected agents vary in cost; Innovar[R] and fentanyl are the most expensive. A 2 ml ampoule of Innovar[R] costs $1.80; 5 ml costs $2.80. Fentanyl, 2 and 5 ml, costs $0.94 and $1.47, respectively. Meperidine (150 mg) and morphine (15 mg) cost $0.30. In many cases nitrous-narcotic-relaxant technique offers minimal cost saving over the inhalation technique.

TOXICITY

We will discuss here the subacute type of toxicity that occurs 2 to 7 days postoperatively. Most of this toxicity of volatile anesthetics is probably secondary to biotransformation. Biotransformation of the volatile anesthetic agents occurs via normal or abnormal (qualitative and/or quantitative) metabolic pathways which may result in viscerotoxicity.

There are predictable animal models for some viscerotoxic manifestations, namely that of methoxyflurane, where the inorganic level of fluoride is directly related to predictable nephrotoxicity. Halothane although definitely capable of causing liver damage is not nearly so predictable in its effect. Reported incidences of liver damage with halothane vary from 1 in 10,000 to 1 in 100,000 administrations. There is evidence that repeated administrations, certain age groups (middle age) and other demographic data (obesity) may be helpful in predicting which patients are at risk to develop hepatotoxicity from halothane. Nevertheless, halothane is a very safe anesthetic agent overall.

Although we know that a level of greater than 80 μM/l of inorganic fluoride in plasma can be associated with nephrotoxicity, these levels are usually not achieved following routine use of enflurane. Enzyme inducing agents such as phenobarbital and phentoin (Dilantin) may cause increased biotransformation of anesthetics by various organs, particularly the liver. This increase in biotransformation may contribute to formation of toxic metabolic products or reactive intermediates and lead to organ damage. Additionally, there may be genetically controlled factors which regulate whether or not patients metabolize halogenated anesthetics via normal or abnormal pathways. Fat serves as an anesthetic reservoir and can continue to release anesthetics for biotransformation for a long period after the cessation of anesthetic administration. Thus, the total dose of anesthetic administered is important, as excess anesthetic will end up in adipose tissue. It is recognized that the obese patient biotransforms more inhalation anesthetic than the svelte one.

On the other end of the spectrum, injected anesthetics are most likely to have toxicity secondary only to overdosage, that is, pharmacologic extensions of activity. Nitrous oxide has been shown to be an immunosuppressive agent. Toxicity due to nitrous oxide consists of environmental pollution (operating room contamination) with trace amounts of nitrous oxide. This "toxicity" can be eliminated by scavenging waste gases in the operating room. Overall, viscerotoxicity is probably a much greater consideration for the inhaled than for the injected agents.

Many anesthesiologists refrain from using halogenated agents because they wish to protect themselves medicolegally from the potential of organ toxicity. I do not feel that this necessarily represents good practice. It would be far better for the anesthesiologist to consider an *indication* for each anesthetic agent administered rather than looking specifically for contraindications. If an anesthesiologist feels that a halogenated anesthetic agent is the anesthetic of choice for a particular patient, he should not be swayed by the potential of viscerotoxicity unless dealing with a patient in a high risk category for development of that complication. A preoperative note indicating reason for selection of a particular anesthetic is valuable in this regard.

CARDIOVASCULAR EFFECTS

The cardiovascular system is influenced by both volatile agents and injected anesthetics. As a general rule, the injected anesthetics are less depressing to the cardiovascular system than are the volatile halogenated anesthetics. The drop in blood pressure seen following administration of inhalation agents is usually corrected by surgical stimulation or adequate fluid load. Surgical stimulation during anesthesia with nitrous-narcotic-relaxant technique frequently causes undesirable elevations of blood pressure. This is due to the sympathetic nervous system stimulation (catecholamine release) effect of surgery. The halogenated agents decrease cardiac output to a greater degree than do the injectable agents. Obviously, the induction of anesthesia is the most hazardous event because with surgical stimulation cardiac output may return to normal levels. An interesting sidelight in this regard is ketamine. *In vivo* ketamine stimulates the cardiovascular system but is a negative inotropic drug in isolated heart preparations. It must be remembered that cardiovascular depression is dose-related with virtually any anesthetic agent that we use.

The decision as to which way the blood pressure is going to go and whether this will or will not be detrimental to the patient is a clinical judgement. The general cardiovascular status of the patient, his blood volume, and his age are all important factors to be considered. Ideally, most patients undergoing surgery on an outpatient basis are free of cardiovascular disease. An occasional treated hypertensive patient is seen in the outpatient setting. In these patients better control of the blood pressure would probably be obtained with use of an inhaled volatile anesthetic agent rather than injectable anesthetics.

Cardiac arrhythmias are more commonly seen with volatile agents than with intravenous agents. The cardiac rhythm in conjunction with vasopressors, particularly epinephrine, is more stable with injected than inhaled anesthesia. About 2 or 3 μg/kg of epinephrine causes ventricular extrasystoles during halothane anesthesia. Although the epinephrine arrhythmia threshold with enflurane is $2^1/_2$ times greater than with halothane, it is still far less than with injected agents. In most instances, the amount of epinephrine injected clinically is well below the arrhythmia threshold of all anesthetics. It is my opinion that the risk of arrhythmias should be reduced whenever possible. Pertinent literature recommends an upper limit of 100 μg of epinephrine (in an average adult) in any 10-minute period during halothane anesthesia. Nitrous-narcotic-relaxant or enflurane anesthesia would certainly be my choice were I certain that the surgeon was going to inject epinephrine.

RESPIRATORY EFFECTS

Respiratory depression is produced almost equally with both anesthetic techniques (injected or inhaled). All anesthetic agents discussed here are respiratory depressants measured by changes in the carbon dioxide response curve. Depression of respiration at lighter levels of anesthesia is counteracted by surgical stimulation, especially with halogenated agents. Spontaneous ventilation can be employed with both inhaled and injected agents provided neuromuscular blocking drugs are not used. Nevertheless, the halogenated agents lend themselves more easily to spontaneous ventilation technique.

NEUROMUSCULAR BLOCKING AGENTS

Neuromuscular blocking agents are used quite frequently in outpatient anesthesia. I will not discuss single dose succinylcholine for endotracheal intubation either with or without pretreatment with a nondepolarizer. For anesthetics of short duration, succinylcholine by dilute infusion is an excellent way to provide muscle relaxation. If the anesthetic is expected to last longer than 45 minutes, a better choice would be a small dose of a nonpolarizating neuromuscular blocker (d-tubocurarine, gallamine, or pancuronium). The halogenated anesthetic agents potentiate the nondepolarizating neuromuscular blockers to a greater extent than do injected agents, allowing a smaller dosage of relaxant to be used. Regardless of whether injected or inhaled agents are used, neuromuscular blockers should not be administered unless monitored with a peripheral nerve stimulator. At the conclusion of anesthesia, sustained tetanus for 5 seconds in response to 50 or 100 Hz stimulation will assure normal neuromuscular transmission. The new stick-on electrodes have eliminated the invasiveness of this monitoring technique; the leads can be comfortably applied while the patient is awake.

RECOVERY ROOM

Postoperative events occurring after the anesthetic is terminated are very important in the outpatient. Inhaled anesthetics with low solubility have an effect that dissipates very rapidly. With injected agents the effects linger longer. There is the possibility of recovery room depression, primarily from "renarcotization." The use of a short-acting narcotic (fentanyl) can minimize renarcotization. It is important to realize that morphine and meperidine have a duration of action longer than that of naloxone. As stated previously, *intramuscular* naloxone must be administered in order to prevent recurrent respiratory depression from the narcotic. Even with short-acting narcotics there is a slight rightward shift in the carbon dioxide response curve 1 to

2 hours after the operation is completed, and a potential for respiratory depression in the recovery room exists.

It must be emphasized that all anesthetics demand and deserve adequate postoperative monitoring. The real "bottom line" with regard to outpatient anesthesia is: "When can the patient be safely discharged from the recovery room?" Innovar[R] should be used very cautiously in outpatients as the tranquilizing component (droperidol) has a relatively long half-life (6 hours). Some pain in the postoperative period is probably a beneficial phenomenon for overcoming depressant effects of anesthetics. Its presence probably allows patients to be discharged from the recovery room at the earliest possible time. There is less postoperative pain relief afforded by the inhalation agents than by the injected agents because of their evanescent duration. It is my opinion (supported by clinical impressions) that patients "go home" after outpatient anesthesia equally rapidly with inhaled or injected agents provided the agents are administered properly.

AWARENESS

Awareness during anesthesia is a concern of the anesthesiologist both medicolegally and from an aesthetic and moral standpoint. With the inhaled anesthetic agents, if there is lack of movement in response to a painful stimulus the patient almost always has amnesia/hypnosis. Additionally, it is easy to tie the depth of anesthesia to an inhaled concentration for each inhalation agent. Although we routinely give nitrous-narcotic-relaxant anesthesia without patient awareness, the potential for awareness is always paramount to the anesthesiologist. Barbiturates produce excellent amnesia and hypnosis, as does diazepam. Unfortunately diazepam and Innovar[R] have pharmacologic half-lives not well suited to use in the outpatient setting. Therefore, narcotics and barbiturates are the standbys for producing amnesia, sedation, and hypnosis in the adult surgical outpatient with the nitrous-narcotic-relaxant technique.

SKILL AND LIMITATION IN TECHNIQUE

The skill of the anesthesiologist and the potential for human error are important considerations in evaluating nitrous-narcotic-relaxant anesthesia vs. the inhalation agents. A number of injections must be given frequently during the nitrous-relaxant technique. Thus, the possibility exists of inadvertently injecting a medication at the wrong time. It is my opinion that a greater degree of consummate skill is required to perform intravenous anesthesia vs. inhaled anesthesia. Part of this is due to the potential for human error and part to limitation of the technique. For a relatively unskilled person, inhalation anesthesia is probably a better choice. Unskilled persons should not become overconfident in the use of injected anesthesia, thinking that they can "bail out" using antagonist drugs.

High altitudes with barometric pressures less than 600 torr limit the effective use of nitrous oxide.

MISCELLANEOUS

A stiff chest ("wooden rigidity") can result from the rapid injection of narcotics. This is most frequently seen with the rapid injection of Innovar[R] or fentanyl. These drugs should be injected slowly to minimize this effect. A stiff chest can decrease the functional residual capacity and increase the tendency toward airway closure with shunting and ventilation-perfusion abnormalities with resulting low arterial oxygen tensions. This is especially true in the absence of neuromuscular blockers. If neuromuscular blockers are used, the stiff chest should not represent a significant problem.

Most of the inhaled anesthetics administered in the outpatient setting are given by a mask rather than through an endotracheal tube. It is my opinion that volatile anesthesia is easier to administer with a mask than is nitrous-narcotic-relaxant anesthesia. If an endotracheal tube is to be used, however, this difference is eliminated.

SUMMARY

A review of the advantages and disadvantages of nitrous-narcotic-relaxant vs. inhaled volatile anesthesia for outpatients results in the following conclusion: For most anesthesiologists in most settings, inhaled volatile anesthesia (with or without supplemental neuromuscular blocking agents) is probably superior to nitrous-narcotic-relaxant anesthesia (Table 1). Every

Table 1. Nitrous-Narcotic vs. Volatile Anesthetics.

Criteria	*N_2O-Narcotic*	*Volatile Agents*
Retrievability and control	−	++
Cost	+	0
Toxicity	++	−
Cardiovascular effects	0	−
Respiratory effects	0	0
Muscle relaxation and relaxant	0	+
Recovery room	−	+
Awareness	−	+
Skill and technique limitations	−	+
Miscellaneous	0	0

+ = advantage   − = disadvantage   0 = not a factor

anesthesiologist administering anesthesia to adult surgical patients on an outpatient basis must evaluate the surgical procedure being performed and his own anesthetic skill in deciding which of these techniques is best suited to any particular patient. It is only by constant attention to all factors that we can continue to provide the finest in anesthetic care for adult outpatients.

REFERENCES

1. Eger, E. I., II: *Anesthetic uptake and action.* Williams and Wilkins Company, Baltimore, 1974.
2. Brown, B. R., Jr.: *Clinical significance of the biotransformation of inhalation anesthetics.* South. Med. J. 69:554–556, May 1976.
3. *Anesthesia: inhaled or injected.* Parts I and II, Ohio Medical Products, 1977.
4. Miller, R. D.: *Antagonism of neuromuscular blockade.* Anesthesiology 44:318–329, April 1976.
5. Miller, R. D., Way, W. L., Dolan, W. M., et al.: *The dependence of pancuronium and d-tubocurarine induced neuromuscular blockades on aveolar concentrations of halothane and Forane.* Anesthesiology 37:573–581, December 1972.
6. Cullen, D. J., Eger, E. I., II, and Stevens, W. C.: *Clinical signs of anesthesia.* Anesthesiology 36:21–36, January 1972.
7. Eger, E. I., II, Smith, N. T., Cullen, D. J., et al.: *A comparison of the cardiovascular effects, halothane, fluroxene, ether and cyclopropane in man.* Anesthesiology 34:25–31, January 1971.
8. Munson, E. S., Larson, C. P., Badad, A. A., et al.: *The effects of halothane, fluroxene, and cyclopropane on a ventilation: a com-*

parative study in man. Anesthesiology 27:716–728, November–December 1966.

9. Brown, B. R., Jr., and Crout, J. R.: *A comparative study of the effects of five general anesthetics on myocardial contractility: I. isometric conditions.* Anesthesiology 34:236–245, March 1971.
10. Bahlman, S. H., Eger, E. I., II, Halsey, M. J., et al.: *Cardiovascular effects of halothane in man during spontaneous ventilation.* Anesthesiology 36:494–505, May 1972.
11. *A symposium on enflurane.* Acta Anesthesiol. Belg. 25:169–299, March 1974.
12. Fogdall, R. P., and Miller, R. D.: *Neuromuscular effects of enflurane, alone and combined with d-tubocurarine, pancuronium, and succinylcholine in man.* Anesthesiology 42:173–178, February 1975.
13. Becker, L. D., Paulson, B. A., Miller, R. D., et al.: *Biphasic respiratory depression after fentanyl-droperidol or fentanyl alone used to supplement nitrous oxide anesthesia.* Anesthesiology 44:291–296, April 1976.
14. Johnston, R. R., and Eger, E. I., II: *A comparative interaction of epinephrine with halothane, enflurane and isoflurane in man.* Abstracts of scientific papers, 1974 Annual meeting, American Society of Anesthesiologists, pp. 53–54.

6

AN OUTPATIENT PAIN SERVICE

Donald E. Howland, M. D., and
Laurel Ann Howland, R. N.

For manifold reasons, most anesthesiologists in private practice have an aversion to pain therapy. Dr. Donald Howland, a practitioner associated with the Phoenix Surgicenter[R], describes a successful and gratifying private practice pain clinic. As anesthesiologists we possess skills in pain management that can be employed outside the operating room environment, and which are not possessed by other specialties. Chronic pain problems constitute a deviation from an otherwise excellent standard of health care delivery in the United States. Recent statistics indicate that there are approximately seven million people in this country who are totally or partially disabled by chronic low back and neck pain alone. Most are between 35 and 60 years of age. With so many disabled in the prime of life, the economic effect in terms of jobs abandoned is enormous. This neglected area is a challenge to the anesthesiologist, and one that he must not ignore.

Burnell R. Brown, Jr.

Until recently, little has appeared in medical literature regarding the treatment of pain. Outstanding exceptions, of course, are *The Management of Pain* by Bonica and *Regional Block* by Moore. Over the past few years more articles have been appearing but they deal mostly with university pain clinics and with chronic pain. A great deal of emphasis has been in the area of psychiatric rehabilitation. Evolving from these writings is the promotion of a multidisciplinary approach, which is the greatest breakthrough in care of the patient experiencing pain.

Pain units in large hospitals and university settings are much needed, but the anesthesiologist in private practice can and should play an important role in the "front lines" of pain control. He should, in addition, serve a valuable function as part of the team in the large multidisciplinary centers.

Much of the pain patients endure (acute, acute approaching chronic, and chronic) lends itself to the anesthesiologist's expertise with blocks in both diagnosis and treatment. Active participation of anesthesiologists in any community will prevent many problems from reaching the chronic pain syndrome, and help guide patients back to useful and productive lives.

One of the problems anesthesiologists face is an already overtaxing practice which seems to limit us to the operating, recovery, and intensive care areas of the hospital. We believe there are enough anesthesiologists interested in pain problems and nerve blocks to fill this gap in the private sector of medical care, if these individuals are given but a few simple guidelines and perhaps a little encouragement. Once the word spreads that an anesthesiologist is willing to consult pain problems, his practice will be so rapidly inundated with pain patients that he will have no time available to the OR and will need a second, third, and even fourth person to assist in the pain practice. (The size of this group obviously depends on the size of the community.)

As one becomes more involved in pain problems, the requirements for greater knowledge than just that of nerve blocks becomes apparent. One must become familiar with the psychology of both acute and chronic pain and conversant with other therapeutic modalities such as neurosurgery, orthopedic surgery, physical medicine, and rehabilitation. As a result one develops special acumen in differential diagnosis of pain problems. Avenues of referral in psychology, psychiatry, neurosurgery, orthopedic surgery, neurology, internal medicine, physical medicine, and rehabilitation must be developed. As not all anesthesiologists have enthusiasm or interest in caring for pain problems, so this disinterest holds true among some in the other specialties. Physicians with firm commitment to and interest in pain must be sought out. As this consultative structure becomes manifest, what has indeed evolved? A loosely knit, but effective, multidisciplinary pain clinic for outpatient care. This occasionally leads to hospital care, psychiatric and otherwise, of a certain percentage of the patient load. It certainly obviates furtive efforts (surgical, multiple drug, multiple doctors, incompetent care) exerted by and upon those patients. Therefore, anesthesiologists involved with pain problems who are familiar with the psychological, surgical, medical, and rehabilitative treatments available can provide both diagnostic and therapeutic blocks and, in addition, an excellent screening area. The anesthesiologist can develop expertise in other parameters of pain control paralleling his skills. These include transcutaneous nerve stimulators, acupuncture, and perhaps biofeedback and hypnosis.

Initially, many anesthesiologists otherwise interested tend to "back off" because adeptness in performing a myriad of nerve blocks must be developed, and in the beginning failures are discouraging. Persistence and frequent experience will develop one's expertise. If one fails to produce an adequate block, a simple explanation to the patient that "I missed the nerve or didn't get quite enough medicine into it; we'll repeat the anesthesia" will usually suffice to reassure the patient. I have found this explanation to be well accepted in our practice.

The economic feasibility of this kind of practice is also a concern. As one starts, it takes longer to interview, examine, and diagnose the problem. Also, more time is required to perform the block, or other therapy deemed appropriate, and time and dollars become real considerations. As abilities improve and patient load increases (indeed, it will geometrically), the economics of a pain practice become feasible.

The next consideration is the physical facilities and personnel requirements. In most areas, as initially in ours, the only space available for performing diagnostic and therapeutic blocks is the recovery and/or emergency rooms, which rapidly become overtaxed and unable to accommodate the number of patients requiring care. As the patient load grows, administrative officials readily become convinced that a geographic area designed for an outpatient "nerve block/pain care unit" is necessary.

In addition, nursing and administrative personnel are required for safe care of patients, some of whom will receive major nerve blocks with incumbent potential complications. This can be supplied by the hospital administration or by an outside facility. In Phoenix, we have been most fortunate that Dr. Reed of Surgicenter[R] has created such a facility to which all anesthesiologists may bring patients. This facility has proved highly successful and fills a great community need. Over a period of several years, the housing has changed from time to time; it has evolved to a design which encompasses 3,000 square feet (Fig. 1).

One should note that office space is included to allow for outpatient psychological testing and therapy, including biofeedback. Physician office space is contingent to, but separated from, the treatment area. Two "nerve block" rooms and a recovery room, equipped as an OR, occupy the main area. Immediately available to this area are six smaller rooms where patients receiving other modalities of therapy can be cared for. A business office and reception area are located at the entrance with a good patient traffic pattern. The business office houses the receptionist-stenographer/secretary and the accounting department.

In our estimation, it is imperative that all patients be seen on a physician referral basis only. This provides one with an initial medical work-up to serve as a springboard for final examination and evaluation. In this way, the anesthesiologist's time is used in the most efficient manner.

If appointments are made far enough in advance, the patient is provided the following questionnaire to complete at his leisure at home. If such is not the case, the patient completes the form on admission to the unit.

Our unit employs four nurses who are specially selected. Each has a recovery or ICU background and is of the temperament to supply this special category of patient the appropriate psychological support. In addition, by association and special study, including medical meetings highlighting topics on pain problems, the nurses have developed a keen awareness of the

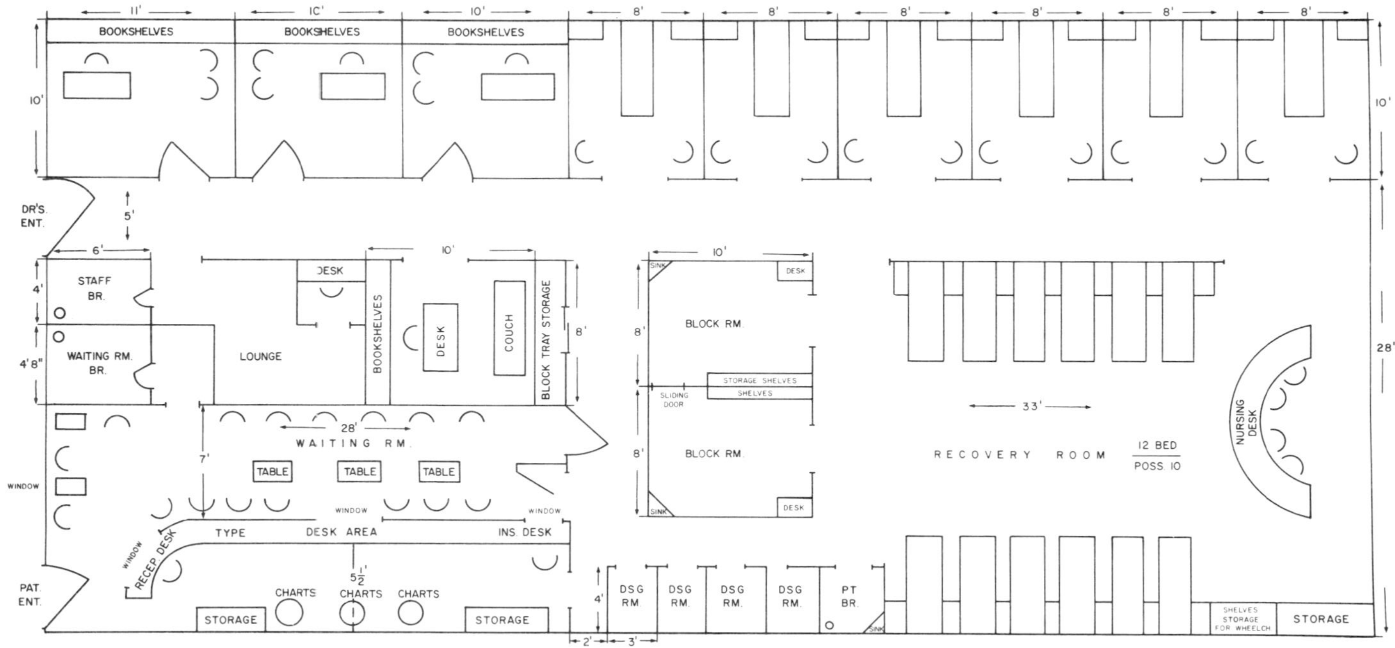

FIGURE 1. Schematic drawing of the Surgicenter[R], Phoenix.

MEDICAL INFORMATION

PLEASE READ THESE SHEETS CAREFULLY AND ANSWER ALL QUESTIONS TO THE BEST OF YOUR ABILITY.

A. NAME____

(LAST) (FIRST) (MIDDLE INITIAL)

AGE____________ HEIGHT____________ WEIGHT____________

REFERRING PHYSICIAN(S) ____________ OTHER PHYSICIANS SEEN FOR YOUR PAIN PROBLEM:

____________ ____________

____________ ____________

B. ALLERGIES____________ REACTIONS____________

____________ ____________

____________ ____________

C. PLEASE CIRCLE APPROPRIATE DESCRIPTION OF YOUR PAIN THEN SHADE IN AREAS THAT YOU HAVE PAIN.

RIGHT

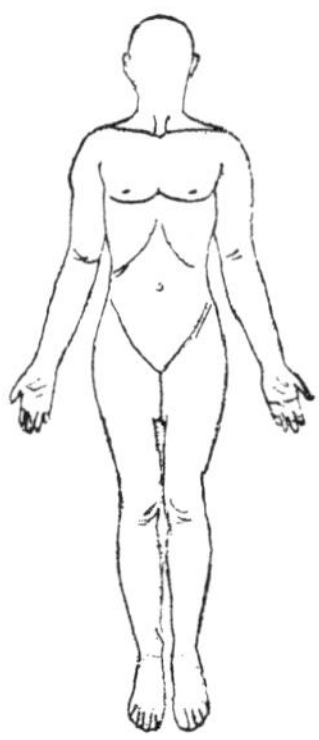

LEFT

THROBBING

ACHING

SHARP

DULL

SHOOTING

TINGLING

BURNING

NUMBNESS

HOTNESS

COLDNESS

CONTINUOUS

INTERMITTENT

LEFT

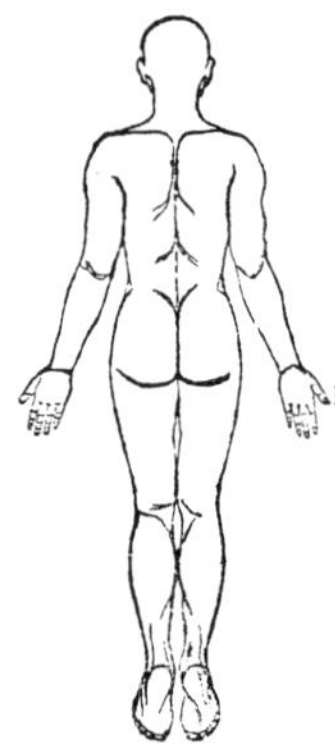

RIGHT

D. DO YOU EVER NOTICE A DIFFERENCE BETWEEN THE TEMPERATURE OF YOUR FEET AND/OR HANDS.

HANDS________ ________ FEET________ ________

YES NO YES NO

E. IS YOUR PAIN THE RESULT OF AN ILLNESS? ______ ______ DATE(S)__________________
YES NO

PLEASE EXPLAIN ____

F. IS YOUR PAIN THE RESULT OF AN ACCIDENT? ________ ________ DATE(S)______________
YES NO

PLEASE EXPLAIN____

G. HOW LONG HAVE YOU HAD THIS PAIN?____

H. ARE YOU EVER PAIN FREE?________ ______
YES NO

PLEASE EXPLAIN____

I. IF YOUR PAIN IS INTERMITTENT, HOW LONG DO EPISODES LAST?______________________

J. DOES COUGHING, SNEEZING OR STRAINING INCREASE YOUR PAIN?_______ _______
YES NO

K. DOES EATING INCREASE YOUR PAIN?______ ______
YES NO

L. DOES ACTIVITY AFFECT YOUR PAIN? _______ _______
YES NO

PLEASE EXPLAIN____

M. ARE YOU ACTIVE DURING THE DAY? ______ ______
YES NO

IF YES, HOW LONG CAN YOU TOLERATE BEING UP DURING THE DAY?___________________

N. WHAT ACTIVITIES DO YOU ENJOY?____

O. IS IT NECESSARY FOR YOU TO REST DURING THE DAY________ ________
YES NO

IF YES, HOW LONG_________________

P. HOW MANY HOURS DO YOU SLEEP AT NIGHT____________________ DAY_____________

Q. DOES YOUR PAIN AFFECT YOUR SLEEP? ________ ________
YES NO

R. PLEASE CHECK ANY OF THE TREATMENTS YOU HAVE HAD, PLEASE INCLUDE DATES AND RESULTS IF POSSIBLE.

TREATMENTS	YES	NO	DATE DONE	DID THIS HELP YOUR PAIN? YES	NO
NERVE BLOCKS	___	___	_________	_______	_______
NERVE STIMULATOR (NEURO PAC)	___	___	_________	_______	_______
PHYSICAL THERAPY	___	___	_________	_______	_______

HEAT TREATMENTS	___	___	________	______	______
MASSAGE	___	___	________	______	______
TRACTION	___	___	________	______	______
ACUPUNCTURE	___	___	________	______	______
CHIROPRACTIC	___	___	________	______	______
OTHER					
________________	___	___	________	______	______
________________	___	___	________	______	______

R2. PLEASE INDICATE IF YOU HAVE HAD ANY OF THESE PROCEDURES AND THE DATES IF POSSIBLE

	YES	NO	DATE		YES	NO	DATE
X-RAY	______	______	________	MYELOGRAM	______	______	______
EMG	______	______	________	DISCOGRAM	______	______	______

S. PLEASE LIST ALL MEDICATIONS YOU ARE NOW TAKING, PLEASE INCLUDE DR. PRESCRIBING PRESCRIPTIONS IF POSSIBLE.

MEDICATION	DESCRIPTION (i.e. Color tab, or capsule, etc.)	TAKEN FOR	HOW OFTEN DO YOU TAKE	PRESCRIBING PHYSICIAN
________	____________	________	________	____________
________	____________	________	________	____________
________	____________	________	________	____________
________	____________	________	________	____________

T. HAVE YOU EVER TAKEN CORTISONE? ______ YES ______ NO

IF SO, WHEN AND FOR WHAT REASON?

DATE	WHAT REASON TAKEN FOR
__________	______________________________
__________	______________________________

U. HAVE YOU EVER BEEN GIVEN A LOCAL ANESTHETIC? ______ YES ______ NO (i.e. Given by a Dentist or Doctor)

IF YES, FOR WHAT REASON?______________________________

V. PLEASE LIST ANY SERIOUS ILLNESSES YOU HAVE OR MAY HAVE HAD. (IN ADDITION TO YOUR PAIN PROBLEM.)

____

____

W. PLEASE LIST ALL SURGERIES YOU HAVE HAD, ALSO DATES AND SURGEON'S NAME IF POSSIBLE.

SURGERY	DATE	SURGEON
____________	________	______________
____________	________	______________
____________	________	______________
____________	________	______________
____________	________	______________

X. ARE YOU PRESENTLY WORKING? _______ YES _______ NO

Y. WHAT IS YOUR USUAL OCCUPATION? ______________________________

Y2. IF YOU ARE NOT WORKING, WHEN WAS YOUR LAST DAY ON THE JOB? ____________ DATE

Z. HAVE YOU DRIVEN YOURSELF TO OUR OFFICE? _______ YES _______ NO

Z2. IS SOMEONE AVAILABLE TO DRIVE YOU HOME? _______ YES _______ NO

PLEASE ADD ANY COMMENTS YOU FEEL WOULD HELP US IN TREATING YOUR CONDITION.

____

____

____

____

____

____

DATE: ____________________

SIGNATURE OF PATIENT: ______________________________

THANK YOU VERY MUCH FOR TAKING TIME TO FILL OUT THIS FORM.

care of these patients. They aid the patient in completing the form and insure greater and more meaningful input. During the admission time, they also frequently perceive and record psychological problems.

Armed with the referral, the information form and some initial impressions from a qualified nursing staff, the anesthesiologist steps in to examine, question further, diagnose the problem, and prescribe appropriate therapy. In cases where there is variance with the referring physician's impressions, or the problem is more complex than it initially seemed, a phone consultation is held with the referring physician and agreement reached as to the planned course of therapy. At this juncture, should the multidisciplinary approach seem appropriate, the consultation channels are opened.

Each referring physician is given a written consultation including therapy and results. These take the form of "interim notes" if therapy becomes prolonged (longer than a few weeks).

The "Pain Unit" supplies the referring physician and patient a focal point and does much to prevent the course of multiple consultations, drugs, and treatments in which the chronic pain patient becomes involved. Acute pain problems can also be adequately cared for. A certain percentage, if not all, of these acute problems might otherwise progress to chronic problems. One must remember that by the time a patient reaches such a unit, the usual modalities of pain control have been tried and proven ineffective.

With the physical space and staff available as described, a patient load of 400 to 600 visits a month can be accommodated comfortably. We have been accumulating data from this private practice based pain unit. These include no double blind or truly scientific studies but do reflect certain facts about the patient population. The statistics regarding results of therapy are based on both the patient's subjective evaluation and the treating physician's evaluation.

The following statistics reflect incomplete figures but involve a large enough sample of patients to be significant. Charts were reviewed from July of 1973 to July of 1976. These figures were produced on an annual basis, and as one compares the figures year to year, a remarkable closeness pervades, demonstrating reproducibility of results.

In general, the following breakdown of patients occurs (exclusive of low back-sciatic pain patients):

Male 55%
Female 45%
Private insurance 70%
Industrial 30%
Drop out 11%
Referred for psychiatric care 4%
Referred for other medical care 4%
Patients taking potent narcotics and/or tranquilizers on admission 50%
Under 24 years of age 2%
25 to 50 years 47%
50 to 64 years 36%
65 and over 15%

Intercostal neuritis (mostly postoperative).
70% success (75% to 100% remission)
30% failure (less than 75% remission)

These patients were treated with a series of intercostal blocks (3 to 8) which included small amounts of steroid following the initial diagnostic block.

In our unit, when neurolytic blocks seem indicated, we have used 10 percent ammonium sulphate with a 70 percent success rate. We have no incidence of postinjection neuritis as a complication. Our routine has also included a series of three such blocks as we have found one or two injections to be inadequate and feel that more than three add nothing in the face of failure. These are given on an every-other-day basis. The patient is first given an intercostal block as far posterior as possible with lidocaine. After analgesia is established, the ammonium sulphate is injected anterior to the block sight. A 30 percent failure rate with this technique certainly leaves something to be desired. We find ourselves now more inclined toward phenol 6 percent in saline for neurolytic intercostal blocks.

Myofascial syndrome.
75% 75% to 100% pain remission
25% less than 75% pain remission

Therapy for this condition involves trigger point injections with bupivacaine and small amounts of water soluble steroid (e.g. dexamethasone).

Occipital neuritis.

70% 75% to 100% pain remission

30% less than 75% pain remission

This condition almost always involves cervical myofascial problems; therefore, trigger points are injected in addition to the occipital nerve blocks. Many of these, of course, are "whiplash" injury patients. We have had about equal success in treating these patients with acupuncture.

Lumbar sympathetic dystrophy.

In this category 40 percent of the patients proved not to have the condition on diagnostic block and 10 percent had elements of dystrophy in their pain complex. The remaining 50 percent responded well to a series of blocks. A very small number of these proved to require surgical or neurolytic intervention. If a patient has not responded with cure in a series of seven or eight blocks, we then resort to destructive procedures. The traditional idea that three blocks should be curative is fallacious. The blocks must also be given in close sequence (2 to 3 times a week). The same is true with stellate ganglion blocks.

Stellate dystrophy.

Here 25 percent proved not to have the condition on diagnostic block, and 15 percent proved to have elements of dystrophy in their pain complex. Sixty percent responded well to a series of blocks.

Herpes zoster.

This condition has proved an enigma over the years, and our success in its treatment until the past 18 months had been a disappointing 25 to 30 percent.

Using the following method, we have achieved an 85 to 100 percent success rate. Treatment of acute herpes with sympathetic blocks (again in close order—2 or 3 per week) results in accelerated drying of the lesions and remission of pain after three or four blocks. There is also no evidence at present of any occurrence of postherpetic pain following such blocks. The thoracic and upper lumbar areas might be treated in the same fashion with epidural blocks with dilute solutions for sympathetic blockade, but we have not attempted this on outpatients.

If the lesions in the acute phase are not applicable to stellate or lumbar sympathetic blocks, or the patient is suffering postherpetic pain, intracutaneous and subcutaneous infiltration of the involved area with bupivacaine .05 percent and Kenalog will produce excellent results.

The ratio we use, recommended by Dr. Frank Moya, is 10 ml 0.5 percent bupivacaine with 5 mg Kenalog. A sufficient amount should be used to infiltrate the involved area (often 30 to 40 ml). This technique, used on a weekly basis, will in 85 to 90 percent of cases completely alleviate the pain (and in acute cases dry up the lesions) in four to six treatments. We inject the acute cases more frequently, every 4 to 5 days, for the initial two to three treatments. Postherpetic pain of 5 years' duration has responded well to this therapy. The success rate in treatment of this condition is a major breakthrough in pain therapy.

Patients suffering back pain are seen in greater numbers than are other pain problems. The general statistics on these patients are:

Male 60%
Female 40%
Private Insurance 65%
Industrial 35%

It is interesting to note that 70 percent of the private patients experienced a 50 percent or greater pain reduction, as did 60 percent of the industrial patients. This presents a significant percentage difference, but not of the magnitude suspected by many.

Drop out 7.5%
Referred for psychiatric care 4.3%
Patients taking potent narcotics and/or tranquilizers 65%
Under 24 years of age 4%
25 to 50 years 56%
50 to 64 years 28%
65 and over 12%

Differential spinal anesthesia is performed initially when we or the referring physician are suspicious of the patient's complaint. A certain number of patients not responding to treatment as expected, or coming under psychiatric suspicion, are also provided this technique. Interestingly, of patients in these categories, 80 percent were referred for psychiatric evaluation.

The following figures are of some interest. It is our feeling that treatment with epidural steroids produces better results when administered by the caudal route, or a combination of caudal and lumbar routes, as opposed to the lumbar approach alone. These patients are seen once a week for 3 weeks.

Patients with no back surgery:
- Three caudals:
  - 65% 50% or more remission
  - 50% essentially pain free
- Three lumbar epidural blocks:
  - 65% 50% or more remission
  - 30% essentially pain free
- Combination of caudal and lumbar approaches:
  - 70% 50% or more remission
  - 42% essentially pain free

Patients with one back surgery:
- Three caudals:
  - 60% 50% or more remission
  - 30% essentially pain free
- Three lumbar epidurals (very few patients):
  - 40% 50% or more improvement
  - 18% essentially pain free
- Combination of caudal and lumbar epidural:
  - 68% 50% or more improvement
  - 42% essentially pain free

When pain persists and is unilateral, we maintain a high index of suspicion of sympathetic dystrophy. Eighteen percent of the unoperated patients received diagnostic sympathetic blocks, with 58 percent of these being positive. Of those patients having one back surgery, 20 percent were given diagnostic lumbar sympathetic blocks, and of these, 40 percent were positive. These are very significant figures, and demonstrate the necessity that a high index of suspicion be held in caring for these patients.

The scope of this chapter does not allow for a detailed discussion of any specific pain problem. We hope that it will engender interest among anesthesiologists in pain treatment. Our abilities with blocks offer the entree and from there more knowledge and skill must evolve. We strongly encourage our fellow anesthesiologists with an interest in this area to become involved.

REFERENCES

1. Bonica, J. J.: *The management of pain.* Lea & Febiger, Philadelphia, 1953.
2. Moore, D.: *Regional block.* C. C Thomas Co., Springfield, Illinois, 1971.
3. Melzack, R., Stillwell, D. M., and Fox, E. J.: *Trigger points and acupuncture points for pain: correlations and implications.* Pain, Vol. 3, No. 1:3–23, 1977.
4. Brown, B. R.: *Office management of common musculoskeletal pain syndromes.* Fam. Phys., Vol. 6, No. 3:92–98. 1972.
5. Bonica, J. J.: *Symposium on pain: part I.* Arch. Surg., Vol. 112, No. 6:749–788, 1977.
6. Bonica, J. J.: *Symposium on pain: part II.* Arch. Surg., Vol. 112, No. 7:861–902, 1977.
7. Winnie, A. P., and Collins, V. J.: *The pain clinic: 1. differential neural blockade in pain syndromes of questionable etiology.* Med. Clin. North. Am. 52:123–129, 1968.
8. deJong, R. H.: *Neural blockade by local anesthetics.* JAMA 238:1383–1385, 1977.
9. Defalque, R. J.: *The anesthesiologist's role in the management of chronic pain.* Anesth. Rev. 4:19–23, 1977.
10. Bonica, J. J.: *Symposium: considerations in management of acute pain.* Hosp. Pract., January 1977.
11. Winnie, A. P.: *Regional anesthesia.* Surg. Clin. North Am., Vol. 55, 861–892, 1975.
12. Winnie, A. P., Murthy, R., and Durrani, Z.: *Pharmacologic reversal of Horner's syndrome following stellate ganglion block.* Anesthesia, Vol. 41, 615–617, December 1974.
13. Winnie, A. P., Hartman, J. T., and Meyers, H. L., Jr.: *Pain clinic II, intradural and extradural cortical steroids for sciatica.* Anesth. Analg. (Cleve), Vol. 51, 990–1003, November–December 1972.
14. Winnie, A. P., Hartman, J. T., and Meyers, H. L., Jr: *Inguinal paravascular technique of lumbar plexus anesthesia: the three in one block.* Anesth. Analg. (Cleve), Vol. 52, 989–996, November–December 1973.

15. Winnie, A. P., Hartman, J. T., and Meyers, H. L., Jr.: *Interscalene cervical plexus block: a single injection technique.* Anesth. Analg. (Cleve), Vol. 54, 370–375, May–June 1975.
16. Carron, H., Litiviller, R.: *Stellate ganglion block.* Anesth. Analg. (Cleve), Vol. 54, 567–570, September–October 1977.
17. Carron, H., and Epstein, B. S.: *Complications of acupuncture.* JAMA, Vol. 228, 1552–1554, June 17, 1974.
18. Stilz, R. J., Carron, H., and Sanders, D. B.: *Reflex sympathetic dystrophy in a six year old: successful treatment of transcutaneous nerve stimulator.* Anesth. Analg. (Cleve), Vol. 56, 438–443, May–June 1977.

7

SPECIAL REGIONAL ANESTHETIC TECHNIQUES IN AMBULATORY ANESTHESIA

Fred H. Landeen, M.D.,
Lloyd Epstein, M.D., and
Lawrence Haas, M.D.

Regional procedures are frequently shunned by anesthetists in the outpatient environment. The reasons are legion but include high failure rate, long recovery room periods for spinal and epidural blocks, and delayed complications of spinal anesthesia, such as headache. However, there is general consensus that for certain procedures, such as upper extremity surgery and perianal surgery in the Buie (prone jack-knife) position, conduction anesthesia has tremendous potential advantages over general anesthesia. One of the problems with the intravenous (Bier) regional technique has been back-bleeding from the wound site. General anesthesia for rectal surgery in the Buie position is the harbinger of potentially frightful physiologic derangements. In the following chapter these problems are reviewed and new solutions presented.

Burnell R. Brown, Jr.

In this chapter, two recently developed areas of conduction anesthesia are examined which can be utilized very effectively in an outpatient surgical unit. In an ambulatory surgical center, there are certain anesthetic techniques which may be unacceptable for a variety of reasons, either to the patient, the anesthesiologist, or the surgeon. Among the unacceptable techniques are spinal, epidural, caudal, and certain major peripheral nerve blocks. The reasons for unacceptability include time factors such as latency period, high failure rate, or postanesthesia problems, for example postspinal headache.

PERIANAL BLOCK

Rectal surgery on an outpatient presents challenging anesthetic problems. Spinal and caudal anesthesia, the mainstays of the hospital-based patient for proctologic surgery, have obvious shortcomings precluding use. The popular Buie (prone jackknife) position imposes serious physiologic derangements on the patient undergoing general anesthesia. A satisfactory solution has been found in the perianal infiltration block, used by us for classic hemorrhoidectomy, cryohemorrhoidectomy, and fistulectomy and fissure repair.

Preanesthetic Preparation

All patients are admitted to the ambulatory surgery unit 1 hour prior to surgery. They are, of course, NPO. The patient is not premedicated until seen and interviewed by an anesthesiologist.

The anesthetic technique is fully described to the patient, consent signed and the patient moved to the operating room. The patient is placed in a prone position, an intravenous infusion started in the hand, and EKG electrodes and blood pressure cuff are placed in position. Premedication prior to the perianal block technique consists of divided (1/2 ml) doses of Innovar to a maximum of 2 ml in the typical adult. The table is flexed so the patient is in a jack-knife (Buie) position. The buttocks are sprayed with tincture of benzoin and 4 inch tape is used to spread the buttocks apart and expose the anus. The gauze pack is placed over the scrotum or vagina, and the anus and perianal area are prepped with Betadine solution.

Anesthetic Technique

A 3 ml syringe is filled with normal saline with benzyl alcohol 0.9 percent as preservative. A 30 gauge needle is attached to the syringe and anesthetic skin wheals are made at the 12-3-6-9 o'clock positions at the vermillion border of the anus. This technique gives instant skin anesthesia and produces far less injection discomfort than if local anesthesia is used. Following this, a 20 ml syringe is filled with the anesthetic of choice and attached to a 22 gauge needle. Our own selection is a 50:50 mixture of lidocaine 0.5 percent and bupivacaine 0.25 percent. To each 60 ml of this mixture, 1 ml Hyaluronidase is added. The needle is inserted through the skin wheals to a maximum depth of 1.5 cm, and 5 ml of the anesthetic mixture deposited after appropriate aspiration. The needle is then withdrawn almost to the skin and directed at an angle of 60 degrees laterally and at a penetrating angle of 25 degrees to a depth of 2.5 cm. Then 2 to 3 ml of the mixture is deposited as the needle is withdrawn to the skin margin. Thus, a total of 10 ml is injected in the perianal area. The needle is then inserted at the 12 o'clock position, at an angle so that it passes under the coccyx, to a depth of 4 cm. As the needle is withdrawn, 10 ml is deposited. The syringe is refilled and the needle inserted at the 9 and 3 o'clock position to a depth of 4 cm perpendicular to the skin. Five milliliters of local anesthetic is injected at each location. The needle is then ranged both up and down at a 45 degree angle and a maximum depth of 4 cm and an additional 2 to 3 ml of the mixture deposited in each angle. At this point, a total of 40 ml has been injected. The needle is then inserted from the 12 o'clock position laterally at 40 degrees and at a penetrating angle of 40 degrees, in depth to 4 to 6 centimeters, and 10 ml of the mixture injected as the needle is withdrawn. This is the most difficult angle of injection, particularly in obese patients. A 3 inch 22 gauge spinal needle may be needed to obtain proper depth. A total of 60 ml local anesthetic is used for the entire procedure. This totals 150 mg lidocaine and 75 mg bupivacaine, far below toxic levels. The anesthesia should be complete by the time the last 10 ml is injected. The anal reflex should be lost and complete relaxation of the anal sphincter should develop within 10 minutes.

Results

To date a total of 576 patients have been anesthetized in our facility using this technique. There has been a high percentage of patient acceptance of the technique. The following illustrates our results:

Number of cases 576
Satisfactory surgical anesthesia 502
Unsatisfactory surgical anesthesia 74

Unsatisfactory cases all required additional local anesthesia because of a quadrant or area that was insufficiently blocked. The additional block was always performed with 1 percent lidocaine with further local infiltration of the unanesthetized area. Following this additional infiltration, all cases were completed with little or no patient discomfort.

No additional Innovar was required beyond the 2 ml total dose in any case. Anesthesia quality was checked by loss of anal reflex first by the scratch test and then by grasping an external hemorrhoid with an Allis clamp, or by grasping all four quadrants with an Allis clamp. No allergic or toxic reactions were seen with this technique.

Discussion

An alternate and acceptable type of anesthesia is presented for anorectal surgery. Excellent patient acceptance, a high degree of success, safety, and rapid discharge are salient features. We feel it is a better technique than general endotracheal anesthesia and should be an acceptable substitute for spinal, epidural and caudal anesthesia for the inpatient and certainly more acceptable for the outpatient undergoing anorectal surgery.

IMPROVED INTRAVENOUS REGIONAL ANESTHESIA FOR SURGERY OF THE HAND, WRIST, AND FOREARM

Intravenous regional anesthesia was described by Bier[1] in 1908. Until the advent of the amide local anesthetics, it never gained popularity because tissue esterases hydrolyzed procaine, producing a block of only short duration. One of the problems frequently voiced by surgeons is so-called "back-bleeding" when the Bier block is used. We wish to present what we consider to be an improved method, *the second wrap technique,* which provides a nearly bloodless operative field, improves anesthesia, diminishes tourniquet pain, and requires no premedication. The method is similar to that used at the Peter Bent Brigham Hospital in Boston.[2]

On January 1, 1975, we initiated a prospective evaluation of this method at the Ambulatory Surgery Center at Tucson Medical Center. We are reporting 300 consecutive anesthetics for upper extremity surgery administered over 24 months. One of us administered 245 of the blocks and the other, an orthopedic and hand surgeon, performed 89 of the surgical procedures. The study involved 3 anesthesiologists and 42 surgeons in all.

Technique

The tourniquet gauge is calibrated daily by mercury manometer and the cuff and all connections are checked prior to each procedure. No preoperative medication is given. The anesthesiologist evaluates and explains the procedure to the patient. In the operating room, intravenous fluids are started in the nonoperative extremity for administration of medication if needed. That arm also has a blood pressure cuff attached for blood pressure monitoring. A two lead continuous electrocardiogram telemetery set is attached to the patient. A padded dual cuff tourniquet is placed on the operative upper arm and attached to a continuous wall outlet gas supply. Both tourniquets are tested and then placed in the off position. A #22 gauge teflon intravenous catheter is inserted in a hand vein on the involved extremity and taped securely. A roll of cast padding is placed in the hand and the extremity is tightly wrapped with a Martin rubber bandage to the bottom of the dual tourniquet while the arm is elevated. The proximal tourniquet is rapidly inflated to at least 100 torr greater than systolic blood pressure. (In a very large, flabby arm the tourniquet may be elevated to 200 torr greater than systolic pressure.) The Martin bandage is removed and, depending on the size of the arm, 30 to 50 ml 0.5 percent lidocaine without preservative is injected into the indwelling hand vein catheter. If the surgical procedure is to be on the hand or wrist, an ordinary Penrose drain tourniquet is placed around the distal forearm proximal to the wrist prior to injection of the anesthetic. The Penrose tourniquet is left in place until approximately 75 percent of the anesthetic solution is injected. The Penrose tourniquet is then removed, and the remaining lidocaine is injected to allow the solution to flow into the forearm. The Teflon catheter is then withdrawn from the hand vein, the arm elevated and pressure applied to the needle puncture site for approximately 1 minute. The extremity is prepared from the fingers to the distal tourniquet and draped so "the second wrap" can be applied under sterile conditions. Either the extremity is left exposed from the fingertips to the elbow, or a sterile stockinette is applied. After draping the extremity, the surgeon places sterile sponges in the hand and tightly wraps the extremity with a sterile Martin bandage to the distal tourniquet. The distal tourniquet and the proximal tourniquet are released briefly and reinflated.

Discussion

It requires approximately 12 to 15 minutes following injection of the anesthetic for satisfactory anesthesia to occur. This is usually the time it takes to prepare and drape the extremity. If the surgery is to begin sooner, it is occasionally necessary for the surgeon to infiltrate the skin when making the incision. The use of the Penrose tourniquet for hand and wrist surgery seems to hasten the onset of block. We feel that this modification distributes the anesthetic more rapidly and completely by encouraging retrograde perfusion of the anesthetic to the operative area. "The second wrap" improves the technique since it facilitates a dry operative field, which is necessary for hand and wrist surgery. "The second wrap" also forces the anesthetic into the periphery of the venous system, which we feel improves the degree of anesthesia. It also forces the anesthetic under the distal tourniquet so that the tourniquet discomfort is less.

No severe anesthetic reaction, operative complication, or nerve injury was seen in this series. The only side effects were transient tinnitus, dizziness, or nausea that occasionally occurred after quick release and reinflation of the tourniquet. If the total tourniquet time is less than 30 minutes, we have minimized the side effects by the following method. The tourniquet is deflated for approximately 15 seconds and reinflated for 30 to 45 seconds. If side effects are observed after the first tourniquet release, the above technique is repeated two to three times. If the tourniquet is to be released before wound closure, the wound is infiltrated with 1 percent lidocaine prior to tourniquet release.

The surgical procedures for which this method was used were: tumors and ganglions, 153; carpal tunnel, 65; tenosynovitis, 22; tendon surgery, 11; trauma, 24; nerve surgery, 12; Dupuytren's contracture, 13; arthritis, 15; elbow surgery, 2; miscellaneous, 13. In the 330 cases there were no failures. Forty-nine patients (15 percent) required an intravenous narcotic (fentanyl) in amounts up to 200 μg during the procedure to relieve either discomfort or anxiety.

Ahern[3] listed among his contraindications for this technique posttraumatic edema or hematoma, obesity, and local anesthetic idiosyncrasy. Our contraindications are: 1) sensitivity or allergy to lidocaine (a rare phenomenon); 2) infections; 3) operative time over 90 minutes; 4) severe hypertension. Arthritis and diabetes are not considered contraindications.

"The second wrap technique" is a reliable and safe method of anesthesia for surgery of the hand, wrist, and forearm.

REFERENCES

1. Bier, A.: *Ueber einen neuen weg localanasthesie en den gleidmassen zu erzeugen.* Arch. Kin. Chir. 86:1007–1016, 1908.
2. Nalebuff, E. A.: Personal communication.
3. Ahern, G. S.: Personal communication.

8

A CHECK LIST OF DRUG INTERACTIONS IN THE OUTPATIENT

Burnell R. Brown, Jr., M.D., Ph.D.

There is little question that the ideal individual for outpatient anesthesia is an ASA Class I patient. However, in many circumstances, ASA Class II patients are quite suitable for ambulatory surgery. Unfortunately, many of the latter patients are in the "gray zone" with regard to anesthesia risk predicated upon health status and current medications. There are also numerous examples of ASA Class I patients on chronic drug therapy, such as with psychotropic drugs. The decision whether to anesthetize these persons or not falls into that nebulous area of clinical judgment of the anesthesiologist and must be decided by a close evaluation of the patient, the anticipated procedure, and the usual variables attending such a situation.

It is the intent of this chapter to focus on prescription drugs commonly administered on a chronic basis, and outline some precautions and points of pharmacologic interest concerned with anesthetic interactions. This list is certainly not complete. Also, this chapter does not purport to be absolute. It must be emphasized that the decision whether or not to anesthetize a patient does not rest entirely with potential hazards of drug interactions, but rather with the complete clinical assessment of the individual patient.

ANALGESICS

Aspirin use carries with it the problem of increased bleeding. It is a wise precaution to order bleeding and clotting and platelet studies in patients on large daily doses of this salicylate. Interactions of aspirin with anesthetics and anesthetic adjuvants have not been demonstrated. Similarly, acetaminophen (Tylenol) has not been implicated in anesthetic drug interactions, but has been shown to produce a slight increase in the hypoprothrombinemic response when used simultaneously with oral anticoagulants.

Codeine, a morphine congener, may delay gastric emptying, thereby increasing the risk of regurgitation. Although many morphine type analgesics interact with CNS and autonomic drugs, outpatient use of codeine should present no problems since the dose used is generally low.[1]

The use of injectable narcotics, particularly meperidine, is to be strictly avoided in patients receiving monoamine oxidase (MAO) inhibitor therapy such as tranylcypromine. Injection of meperidine in these patients has led to rapid onset of convulsions, hyperthermia, and hypertension.[2] Any patient taking a monoamine oxidase inhibitor is best not treated as an outpatient if general or regional block anesthesia is required.

ANTICONVULSANTS

Epilepsy is a symptom, not a disease. Since it represents one of the most common chronic neurologic disorders, the occasion may frequently arise in which the anesthesiologist is called upon to anesthetize a patient with some form of epilepsy as an outpatient for an incidental problem. Drug interactions occurring with anticonvulsants are common, but unfortunately specific interactions with anesthetics and anesthetic adjuvants have not been studied in depth. Phentoin is a well recognized microsomal enzyme inducer. Thus, pharmacologic effects of other rapidly biotransformed drugs may be shortened if a patient has been chronically taking the anticonvulsant. Although this represents no contraindication, the anesthesiologist should be aware that this classic pharmacologic mechanism may be operative if resistance to drugs is observed. Since the rate of biotransformation of inhaled anesthetics is generally of low order contrasted to that of injected drugs, enzyme induction plays no role in resistance to these drugs.

ANTIDEPRESSANTS

The tricyclic antidepressants typified by amitriptyline are commonly prescribed drugs for various states of mental depression. One of the major pharmacologic mechanisms of amitriptyline and others of similar genre is inhibition of norepinephrine uptake at peripheral postganglionic adrenergic nerve endings and within CNS neurons. Thus, many "side effects" or interactions with other drugs are predicated on an extension of this pharmacologic property. The tricyclics also possess anticholinergic activity and thus would be expected to be additive to the effects of muscarinic receptor blockers such as atropine and glycopyrrolate. Patients at risk to such an interaction are older patients with glaucoma, urinary retention, or cardiac disease. Tricyclic antidepressants in large doses may predispose to intraoperative hypotension and ventricular arrhythmias.

Consideration of patients currently receiving MAO inhibitors has already been discussed. This class of drugs, because of various interactions, probably precludes outpatient anesthesia in patients receiving them.

ANTIHYPERTENSIVES

A decade or so ago there was some concern about anesthetizing the treated hypertensive patient. Fears were expressed that antihypertensive drugs put individuals at greater risk for development of profound hypotension during anesthesia; therefore it was suggested that the antihypertensives be discontinued weeks before anticipated surgery. Analysis of available data now strongly indicates that this is fallacious.[3] The treated hypertensive is a far better candidate for surgery than is the untreated one, just as the effectively treated diabetic is a better candidate than the untreated diabetic. It does behoove the anesthesiologist to have intimate knowledge of the pharmacology of the drugs employed. Propranolol is now widely employed for therapy of early essential hypertension. Recent evidence indicates that even the β-adrenergic receptor blockers should be continued up until the day of surgery, providing the indications for use are valid and appropriate. Evidence of bronchiolar constriction should be evaluated in patients on propranolol preoperatively.

Although moderate to severe essential hypertensive patients with demonstrable organ pathology, such as proteinuria, EKG evidence of left ventricular hypertrophy and histories of CVA, are not candidates for outpatient anesthesia, the early, controlled, essential hypertensive patient is often a suitable candidate for minor outpatient surgery. Because of partial sympatholysis it must be remembered that many essential hypertensive patients may require volume replacement with balanced salt solution to a greater extent than normotensive patients.

TRANQUILIZERS-HYPNOTICS

The benzodiazepine group of tranquilizer drugs such as diazepam and chlordiazepoxide now constitute the most widely prescribed drugs in the United States. Do patients treated with such compounds carry additional hazards with regard to anesthesia? Although there is little scientific documentation to answer this question, the general consensus is that aside from some refractoriness to injected hypnotics they do not. High dosages of phenothiazines (e.g. chlorpromazine) used in therapy of major psychosis produce α-adrenergic receptor blockade, but these patients are not reliable candidates for outpatient anesthesia because of the nature of their psychiatric condition.

Many hypnotics (glutethimide, barbiturates, chloral hydrate, alcohol) are enzyme inducing drugs. Thus, some tolerance to injected anesthetic hypnotics may be expected to occur in patients taking these preparations. All in all, however, such drug interactions are benign.

Although this listing is far from complete, it may be used as a practical guide for safe outpatient anesthesia care of the relatively healthy patient who is a candidate for ambulatory care.

REFERENCES

1. Lasagna, L.: *Drug interactions in the field of analgesic drugs.* Proc. R. Soc. Med. 58:978–984, 1965.
2. Landon, D. R., and Milne, M. D.: *Dangers of monoamine oxidase inhibitors.* Br. Med. J. 2:1752–1753, 1962.
3. Crout, J. R., and Brown, B. R., Jr.: *Anesthesia and the hypertensive patient.* Clin. Anesth. 3:152–161, 1969.

9

MONITORING IN OUTPATIENT ANESTHESIA

Lawrence Adler, M.D.

What instrumentation should be used to monitor the outpatient during anesthesia? Does the new generation of electronic instruments replace and supersede the eye and the "finger on the pulse" of the experienced anesthesiologist? Are there established standards of care dictating minimal monitoring in the typical ASA Class I ambulatory surgical patient? Dr. Adler discusses merits and limitations of instruments commonly employed for this category of patient. Many of these are valuable, but machines, however sophisticated, cannot replace the vigilance of the trained anesthesiologist. Monitors are not independent agents but rather are an adjunct to the physician. Interestingly, the membership of the Arizona Society of Anesthesiologists passed a resolution in 1977 advocating the use of the electrocardiogram for all general anesthetics, even those of short duration in the outpatient.

Dr. Adler also discusses a new generation of on-line gas and vapor monitors, which, although not fully developed now, may be extremely useful in the future. When on-line anesthesia gas and vapor detectors become practical and commercially available, the ability to measure concentrations second to second will be a fact. Low flow techniques with inherent properties of economy and reduction of operating room pollutions should prove of great value in the near future. Only time and experience will tell if these electronic wonders can surpass the skill of the trained eye and hand.

Burnell R. Brown, Jr.

INTRODUCTION

Monitoring requirements for outpatient anesthetics obviously parallel the specific needs of the patients and the surgical procedures. There are differences in risk related to the type of surgery and physical status separating outpatients from inpatients. The former group are short and simple procedures in relatively healthy individuals, so that there is rarely a need for invasive monitoring. The placement of intra-arterial blood pressure devices or Swan-Ganz catheters for pulmonary artery and wedge pressure measurements is beyond the scope of even the most aggressive outpatient anesthesia and surgical service.

Monitoring devices used in outpatient surgery must be troublefree and must have simple and fast application to the patient. Each monitoring device must provide pertinent information to guide therapeutic intervention or provide further degrees of patient safety. Outpatient surgery represents a major new development in health care delivery. Traditional operating room monitors must prove their usefulness in this setting.

CARDIOVASCULAR MONITORS

The EKG provides useful information during anesthesia and surgery.[1] EKG monitors utilizing oscilloscopic displays have become an integral part of modern anesthetic delivery. Space limitations dictate that these devices be small in size, attaching to existing equipment whenever possible. Defibrillator and electrosurgical protection circuits are mandatory features for safe operating room use. Isolated EKG detection circuits employing a floating ground system are used to reduce the chance of microshock and electrosurgical burns at the site of the EKG electrodes.

The use of prejelled disposable surface electrodes makes application to the patient quick and easy. In outpatient surgery, a calibrated EKG trace is usually not necessary. Standard lead II is most frequently monitored because it provides good P wave display. A growing number of anesthetists are using a modified lead I with the left arm placed at the 5th intercostal space in the anterior axillary line or at V_5. This configuration is reported to be the most sensitive to ST segment and T wave changes associated with myocardial ischemia.[2, 3] The large signal from this lead requires little or no amplification, which minimizes the effects of low amplitude electrical interference. The EKG provides continuous information about heart rate and rhythm. It must be remembered that presence of an electrical signal does not insure adequate myocardial contractility. Inhalation anesthetics are classic excitation-contraction uncouplers and consequently electrical signals do not correlate with intensity of heart beat.

BLOOD PRESSURE

Since the first use of Riva-Rocci apparatus to record indirect blood pressure during anesthesia and surgery, this measurement has become one of the most universal monitoring techniques used during anesthesia. The traditional blood pressure cuff in combination with a sound transducer has become the cornerstone of cardiovascular monitoring. Newer devices employing microphones and electronic circuitry have challenged this traditional apparatus in recent years. More sophisticated ultrasonic Doppler devices are now frequently employed. These devices have made blood pressure monitoring practical in small children and in those patients in whom blood pressure is difficult to hear.[4, 5, 6] Doppler devices are indispensible for physicians with hearing difficulties. Unfortunately, proper placement of the sensing device is critical and often more time consuming than with the standard cuff. The oscillotonometer, which employs two air chambers in a single cuff, is an alternative not requiring special placement procedures. This device is reported to have increased accuracy at low pressures[7] but is more time consuming because it requires switching from one cuff to another to obtain actual pressure readings. Given experience on the part of the operator, this is not a problem.

Blood pressure information is useful as a guide to the general status of the circulatory system. In the case of potent halogenated anesthetics, the systolic pressure fall is valuable in total assessment of anesthetic depth. Diastolic pressure change is less useful and in the majority of cases parallels changes seen in the systolic pressure.[8] Despite the lack of specificity of the blood pressure measurement and the wide range of acceptable pressures, this measurement has become the core of patient monitoring.

THE PRECORDIAL AND ESOPHAGEAL STETHOSCOPES

Precordial and esophageal stethoscopes are ideal for use during outpatient surgery and anesthesia. They provide continuous information about heart rate, myocardial strength, and respiration. Placement is rapid, easy, and virtually without risk to the patient. The human ear is very sensitive to changes in the sound pattern heard through the stethoscope. Small changes in heart rate, sound intensity, rhythm, or respiration can be picked up quickly before more serious alterations occur.

The esophageal probe is increasing in popularity because of better acoustical properties than those of the precordial stethoscope. The marketplace has recently been flooded with inexpensive disposable esophageal probes, some of which incorporate temperature sensing devices. Some even offer indwelling EKG electrodes.

NEUROMUSCULAR TRANSMISSION

The development of low cost, battery operated nerve stimulators in conjunction with prejelled disposable surface electrodes has revolutionized assessment of myoneural block. The electrodes are usually placed over the ulnar nerve at the wrist and evoked twitch response is used to guide the administration of neuromuscular blockers and to assure adequacy of recovery from these drugs. This information is of utmost importance for the anesthetist in the outpatient surgical unit since relative overdose or inadequate reversal may interfere with efficient operating room utilization. Postoperative mechanical respiration is obviously not a desirable method of terminating an outpatient anesthetic experience. The routine use of nerve stimulators is recommended for all cases where neuromuscular blocking drugs are used other than for intubation of the trachea.

There are several methods of using stimulators to obtain the clinical information. Testing of single twitch response, testing at tetanic frequencies, and the more recent method employing a train of four stimuli all have their advocates. All these methods can provide the vital information for safe, rational use of neuromuscular blockers.[9, 10]

TEMPERATURE MONITORING

Monitoring body temperature during anesthesia is a fairly easy task. Skin, esophageal, rectal, nasal septal and tympanic membrane probes are available in both reusable and disposable forms. The placement and calibration of these devices is both simple and quick. The entity of malignant hyperplexia has pointed out the need for fairly ubiquitous temperature monitoring. The effects of hypothermia, especially in the neonate, are well recognized. Although in the outpatient surgical environment the usefulness of routine temperature monitoring has not been convincingly demonstrated, at this time it is safe to say that temperature monitoring should be employed to a great extent.

OXYGEN ANALYZERS

There are currently two types of oxygen analyzers in use for continuous monitoring during anesthesia. The first type is a fuel cell or battery powered device which uses ambient oxygen to generate electrical current proportional to the amount of oxygen present. This current is usually read directly on a simple meter as percent oxygen. These devices are simple electrically, but the fuel cell has only a 3-month life expectancy when used in the presence of anesthetics.

The second type of analyzer is the Clark electrode or polarographic sensor. This consists of a silver chloride electrode surrounded by electrolyte solution encased in a Teflon membrane. Oxygen diffuses across the membrane and accepts electrons, causing current flow proportional to concentration. This current is measured and read out as percent oxygen. The Clark electrode is more complex electronically and requires batteries for activation of the circuitry.

Both analyzers are affected by humidity. If calibrated in dry gas, they read low when placed in a high humidity atmosphere. When fuel cells become exhausted or the batteries fail in polarographic analyzers, of course, the device produces erroneous readout. Halothane and enflurane in high concentrations can give falsely high O_2 readings with the Clark electrode but at clinical concentrations this effect is usually minimal.

Most manufacturers offer models with alarms which produce audible signals in oxygen atmospheres dangerous to the patient. This type of device offers an additional safety factor when placed in the anesthesia circuit, guarding against the delivery of hypoxic mixtures due to operator error or oxygen supply failure. These devices are essential for safe closed circuit or low flow anesthesia techniques employing nitrous oxide. The adoption of lower gas flows is one viable method of reducing operating room pollution with excess gases and at the same time producing significant cost savings.

The routine use of oxygen monitoring devices for all life support systems is rapidly becoming the standard. In general, both types of analyzers described here function acceptably well. Calibration may be with room air and/or oxygen and is rapid and easy. Maintenance of fuel cells, electrodes, and batteries for these devices is a relatively simple procedure which needs to be done only a few times each year. The devices can normally be attached to existing anesthesia machines without modification.

GAS ANALYSIS

Methods exist for the continuous on-line measurement of all gases and vapors used by the anesthetist. Mass spectroscopy and infrared and ultraviolet absorption techniques are used to make these measurements. Commercially available devices are large, expensive, difficult to calibrate, and unreliable, and are generally not necessary in the outpatient surgical theater.

Exhaled gas and vapor analysis may completely revolutionize anesthesia administration. End tidal gas levels for the anesthetic gases and carbon dioxide accurately reflect arterial blood levels. Closed circuit administration of anesthesia based on accurate anesthetic blood levels is an interesting and potentially useful alternative to conventional high flow techniques. Development of new gas sensors combined with solid state electronics should provide the anesthesia community with a new generation of practical, rugged, and inexpensive gas analysis capable of use in the outpatient surgical unit.

DISCONNECT ALARMS

Hypoxic episodes due to disruption of the anesthesia delivery systems represent an area of preventable morbidity and mortality. At the present time, disconnect alarms are not standard on anesthesia machines and most ventilators. It is generally assumed that careful patient monitoring—the sixth sense of clinical acuity—is sufficient to detect disruption of the anesthetic apparatus. Despite this constant vigilance by anesthetists, disruption of the anesthesia delivery system still occurs too frequently. Dependable disconnect alarms are long overdue on all anesthesia machines.

RESPIRATION MONITORS

Movements of the reservoir bag are often adequate for monitoring rate and depth of respiration during the outpatient anesthesia experience. Mechanical spirometers such as the Wright Ventimeter are convenient for spot checking and quantitating the minute and tidal volumes. Prolonged exposure to high humidity adversely affects performance, precluding continuous use. Accuracy is greatly affected by flow rate due to the high inertia inherent in this type of device. Calibration is not practical between uses, but the device is accurate enough for most measurements.[11]

Changes in rate and depth of ventilation are useful during short cases as a guide to anesthetic drug administration. Devices capable of providing continuous information about rate and depth of respiration should be highly desirable monitors. Pneumotachygraphs using heated wires, thermostats, or resistance elements have been used for this purpose. Accuracy is acceptable for clinical use[12], but they have never achieved great popularity.

Monitors using chest impedence measurements are useful for determining respiratory rate. To date, volume measurements by this method have not been practical. Impedence devices are totally useless when electrosurgical units are used.

Given the available alternatives, spot checking respiratory volumes with a mechanical spirometer is the most reasonable solution for outpatient anesthesia.

THE FUTURE

The outpatient anesthetist can look forward to a host of new electronic devices. Microprocessors, the "computer-on-a-chip," will become as commonplace as the transistor. They will make possible new, sophisticated, inexpensive monitors. Blood pressure cuffs capable of reading out systolic, diastolic, and mean blood pressures with greater accuracy and precision than is possible today will be available soon. EKG monitors will be able to identify dysrhythmias and alert the anesthetist even when the alterations of display are occult. Solid state temperature and pressure clips will soon appear in a new generation of flow meters, respiration monitors, and temperature measuring devices. The biggest challenge of the future will be deciding what is worthy of being monitored in the outpatient undergoing surgery and anesthesia.

REFERENCES

1. Cannard, T. H., Dripps, R. D., Helwig, J., et al.: *The electrocardiogram during anesthesia and surgery.* Anesthesiology 21:194–202, 1960.
2. Kaplan, J. A., and King, S. P.: *The precordial electrocardiographic lead (V_5) in patients who have coronary-artery disease.* Anesthesiology 45:570–574, 1976.
3. Blackburn, H., Taylor, H. L., Okamoto, N., et al.: *The exercise electrocardiogram: a systematic comparison of chest lead configurations employed for monitoring during exercise,* in Karlomen, M., Ed.: *Physical Activity and the Heart.* Charles C Thomas, Springfield, Ill., 1966.
4. Poppers, P. J., Epstein, R. M., and Donham, R. T.: *Automatic ultrasound monitoring of blood pressure during induced hypotension.* Anesthesiology 35:431–435, 1971.
5. Waltemath, C. L., and Preuss, D. D.: *Determination of blood pressure in low-flow states by the Doppler technique.* Anesthesiology 34:77–79, 1971.
6. Kirby, R. R., Kemmerer, W. T., and Morgan, J. L.: *Transcutaneous Doppler measurement of blood pressure.* Anesthesiology 31:86–89, 1969.
7. Von Bergen, F. H., Weatherhead, S., Freloar, A. E., et al.: *Comparison of indirect and direct methods of measuring arterial blood pressure.* Circulation 10:481–490, 1954.

8. Cullen, D. J.: *Interpretation of blood pressure measurements in anesthesia.* Anesthesiology 40:6–12, 1974.
9. Ali, H. H., and Savarese, J. J.: *Monitoring of neuromuscular function.* Anesthesiology 45:216–249, 1976.
10. Miller, R. D.: *Antagonism of neuromuscular blockade.* Anesthesiology 44:318–329, 1976.
11. Nunn, J. F., and Azi-Ashi, T. I.: *The accuracy of the respirometer and ventigrator.* Br. J. Anaesth. 34:422, 1962.
12. Visick, W. D., Fairley, H. B., and Hickey, R. F.: *Evaluation of a new electronic spirometer.* Anesthesiology 34:475–478, 1971.

INDEX